Lesley

Intyre

GERIATRICS

MANAGEMENT OF COMMON DISEASES IN FAMILY PRACTICE

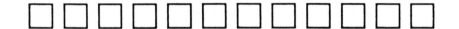

Series Editors: J. Fry and M. Lancaster-Smith

GERIATRICS

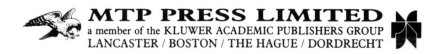

Anthony Martin MD

Consultant Physician, The General Hospital, St Helier, Jersey, Channel Islands; Chairman, The Crawley and Jersey Research Unit

and

Eric Gambrill MB, BS, FRCGP, DRCOG

General Practitioner, Crawley, West Sussex; Associate Adviser in General Practice, South West Thames Region, British Postgraduate Medical Foundation

MTP PRESS LIMITED
a member of the KLUWER ACADEMIC PUBLISHERS GROUP
LANCASTER / BOSTON / THE HAGUE / DORDRECHT

Published in the UK and Europe by
MTP Press Limited
Falcon House
Lancaster, England

British Library Cataloguing in Publication Data

Martin, A.
 Geriatrics.—(Management of common diseases in family practice)
 1. Aged—Diseases
 I. Title   II. Series
 618.97   RC952

 ISBN 0-85200-755-8
 ISBN 0-85200-794-9 Series

Published in the USA by
MTP Press
A division of Kluwer Boston Inc
190 Old Derby Street
Hingham, MA 02043, USA

Library of Congress Cataloging in Publication Data

Martin, Anthony, MD.
 Geriatrics.

 (Management of common diseases in family practice)
 Includes index.
 1. Geriatrics.   I. Gambrill, Eric.   II. Title.
III. Series.   [DNLM: 1. Geriatrics.   WT 100 M379g]
RC952.M364   1986   618.97   86-8367
ISBN 0-85200-755-8

Typeset and printed by
Butler & Tanner Limited, Frome and London

Contents

□ □ □ □ □ □ □ □ □ □ □ □

Series Editors' Foreword	vii
Preface	ix
Acknowledgements	x

Section 1   The Nature of the Problem — 1

Introduction	1
Epidemiology	3
Special factors in the management of disease in the elderly	5
Ageing changes	5
The causes and prevention of disability and disease	7
Attitudes to management	8
Principles of prescribing	9
The nature of some common diseases	10
Organization of care for the elderly	11

Section 2   Symptoms and their Differential Diagnosis — 15

Palpitations	15
Breathlessness	16
Cough	18
Swollen legs	19
'Going off his feet' syndrome	20
Fits, faints and falls	21
Aches and pains	22
Constipation and diarrhoea	23
Failing eyesight and hearing	24
Incontinence	25
Confusion	26

Misery, apathy and sleep problems   28
Collapse   29

Section 3   Specific Disease Complexes   33

Abnormalities of blood pressure   33
Ischaemic heart disease   43
Cardiac dysrhythmias   48
Heart failure   55
Bone disease of ageing   61
Diseases affecting muscles and joints   74
Strokes   84
Parkinsonism and tremor   91
Incontinence   97
The elderly disabled   103
Pain relief   110
Anaemia   114
Thyroid disorders   124
Diabetes mellitus   127
Psychiatric disorders   136

Index   146

Series Editors' Foreword

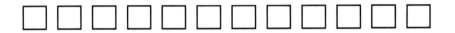

Effective management logically follows accurate diagnosis. Such logic often is difficult to apply in practice. Absolute diagnostic accuracy may not be possible, particularly in the field of primary care, when management has to be on analyis of symptoms and on knowledge of the individual patient and family.

This series follows that on *Problems in Practice* which was concerned more with diagnosis in the widest sense and this series deals more definitively with general care and specific treatment of symptoms and diseases.

Good management must include knowledge of the nature, course and outcome of the conditions, as well as prominent clinical features and assessment and investigations, but the emphasis is on what to do best for the patient.

Family medical practitioners have particular difficulties and advantages in their work. Because they often work in professional islation in the community and deal with relatively small numbers of near-normal patients their experience with the more serious and more rare conditions is restricted. They find it difficult to remain up-to-date with medical advances and even more difficult to decide on the suitability and application of new and relatively untried methods compared with those that are 'old' and well proven.

Their advantages are that because of long-term continuous care for their patients they have come to know them and their families well and are able to become familiar with the more common and less serious diseases of their communities.

This series aims to correct these disadvantages by providing practical information and advice on the less common, potentially serious conditions, but at the same time to take note of the special features of general medical practice.

To achieve these objectives, the *titles* are intentionally those of accepted body systems and population groups.

The *co-authors* are a specialist and a family practitioner so that each can supplement and complement the other.

The *experience bases* are those of the district general hospital and familyu practice. It is here that the day-to-day problems arise.

The *advice and presentation* are practical and have come from many yesrs of conjoint experience of family and hospital practice.

The *series* is intended for family practitioners – the young and the less than young. All should benefit and profit from comparing the views of the authors with their own. Many will coincide, some wil be accepted as new, useful and worthy of application and others may not be acceptable, but nevertheless will stimulate thought and enquiry.

Since medical care in the community and in hospitals involves teamwork, this series also should be of relevance to nurses and others involved in personal and family care.

JOHN FRY
M. LANCASTER-SMITH

Preface

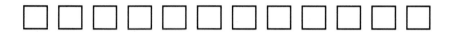

The management of disease in elderly people now constitutes a large part of the general practitioner's workload. The wide spectrum of disease and its co-relation with the degenerative changes that occur with ageing demand great skill of the family physician. Yet, despite this, formal teaching and experience in geriatric medicine has, until very recently, been almost entirely lacking in both pre- and post-registration medical training. It is for this reason that the publishers have asked a specialist physician in geriatric medicine and an experienced general practitioner to combine forces to give some guidance as to how to manage some of the more difficult problems that face those working with the elderly in the community.

Acknowledgements

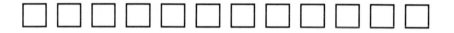

We are grateful to John Fry, general practitioner, Beckenham, Kent, for his unremitting support, encouragement and constructive criticism.

We are also indebted to our many colleagues in both the hospital service and in general practice who continue to stimulate our interest in the problems of the elderly and who endeavour to help us find some of the solutions to them.

Clare Kipping has done a marvellous job typing and word-processing the manuscript. Any errors that remain in the text, however, are entirely our responsibility.

Finally, we thank the publishers for their patience and forbearance during the rather lengthy gestation period of this book.

ANTHONY MARTIN
ERIC GAMBRILL

Section 1

The Nature of the Problem

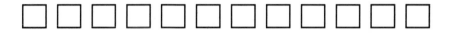

INTRODUCTION

The elderly make up about 14% of the population in Great Britain and number over eight million, of whom about 3.5 million are over 75. These numbers are expected to rise in the next decade and perhaps more significantly the proportion of the elderly population will rise to about 20% of the total (Table 1.1). These trends are mirrored in other Western countries, such as the USA (Table 1.2) and are likely to be even more marked in Oriental countries such as Japan. In Japan there has been a precipitous fall in the birth rate since 1950, which is now the lowest in the world.

Since the elderly are the largest users of health and social services, especially those over 75 years, the impact of this data will not be lost on the health workers and the economists who will know that the generation of the increased reserves needed for the care of the elderly will have to be made by a progressively falling number of employed younger workers.

Table 1.1 The changing population patterns (projected) in the United Kingdom 1983–2011 (Source: OPCS 1983)

Age group (years)	1983	1991	2001	2011
		(millions)		
65–74	4.97	4.99	4.66	4.97
75–84	2.81	3.04	3.05	2.91
85 and over	0.64	0.85	1.05	1.17

Table 1.2 Population projections for the USA 1985–2000 (Source: *International Yearbook* and *Statesman's Who's Who, 1985*)

Age group (years)	1985	1990 (millions)	2000
65–74	16.8	18.0	17.7
75 and over	11.8	13.7	17.3
Total	28.6	31.7	35.0

The need for a better understanding of disease and disability in the old becomes increasingly more urgent in view of their rapidly expanding numbers. Although research into ageing problems and disease in the aged is still in a relatively primitive stage and lags far behind that of the diseases of youth and middle age, great progress has been made in recent years.

The general awareness of the status and contributions of the elderly is, perhaps, beginning to grow again following its great decline in Western communities since the First World War. With it our attitudes to the physical and mental problems of the aged are also beginning to change. In some ways the change in our attitude to the elderly may contribute more than the progress in understanding disease. So much disability in the old is generated by falling social status and the general attitude of the young that the old are 'past it' and not deserving of high technological medicine that it becomes increasingly important to disabuse ourselves of these concepts.

The advances in therapeutics and 'spare part' surgery have been spectacular in the past three decades and it is now possible to provide old people, as well as young, with a greatly enhanced quality of life. Conditions such as osteoarthritis of the hip and severe cardiac conduction disease, to name but two, are now completely remediable by modern technology. Thus, those two conditions, which until recently were often totally crippling, can be ameliorated and enable otherwise fit old people to lead a re-invigorated and independent life.

The appalling consequences of incontinence and depression both for the elderly sufferer and those in his immediate environment can now largely be controlled. The means of control are not always easy and may exercise considerable diagnostic and therapeutic skill. The results of such efforts are very rewarding. No single doctor, nurse, physiotherapist, social worker or housing manager can always hope to achieve many of these aims. A multi-disciplinary approach is essential to the solution of most of the problems of old age. This book, although principally written for doctors, has been written for all those interested in helping with the problems of the elderly, whether professional workers or not.

EPIDEMIOLOGY

Vascular diseases, both of the heart and great arteries, as well as of smaller vessels, are present in the vast majority of the elderly, whether they are symptomatic or not. At least 50% of all those over 65 years will have significant coronary artery disease. Thus the incidence of clinical angina and myocardial infarction can be expected to be much more frequent in this age group than in those who are younger. Strokes, whether a result of cerebral artery thrombosis or, more commonly, emboli from the heart, aorta and carotid/vertebral arteries, are a major cause of death and disability in the old. Arteriosclerotic changes in the abdominal aorta and ilio-femoral tree produce claudication in the mesenteric territory, as well as compromised circulatory changes in the legs, with increasing frequency as age advances. Small vessel disease is most frequently seen in the feet, but may also affect other organs, such as the kidney and gut. Although these small vessel problems are much more frequently seen in those suffering from maturity-onset diabetes, they may occur in the absence of underlying disease.

Cardiac arrhythmias in the elderly are becoming increasingly well-recognized and contribute significantly to both morbidity and mortality. Atrial fibrillation occurs in at least 12% of all aged over 70 years. Atrial fibrillation is a feature of disordered function of the sino-atrial (SA) node: it forms part of the so-called sick sinus syndrome (SSS). Although atrio-ventricular (AV) node disease has been easily identified for a long time, because it causes major symptoms of Stokes–Adams attacks, it is actually much less common than SA node disease. The increasing recognition of conduction tissue disease in the heart is leading to a great increase in pacemaker (PM) implantation in the elderly. The incidence of other arrhythmias in the elderly, such as ventricular premature complexes (VPCs), also increases with age. Although not proven, it is likely that the occurrence of significant numbers of VPCs is associated with an increased likelihood of mortality.

Hypertension in younger life undoubtedly contributes significantly to later life vascular disease, but in a previously normotensive person, the finding of elevated levels of blood pressure in the elderly person may well not have the same significance as in their younger counterparts. Although there is a linear relationship of increasing levels of systolic blood pressure to the incidence of cardiovascular mortality and strokes at all ages, the evidence that this is significant in the elderly is much less strong than in

3

young and middle-aged persons. Thus, although the finding of elevated levels of systolic blood pressure in the elderly is extremely common the clinical significance of this fact is still under considerable discussion.

Musculo-skeletal problems will be one of the most frequent reasons for elderly people to visit their family doctor. Many of these problems will be similar to those of the younger people who make such great demands in primary health care – backache, strained ligaments and painful joints. However, all these problems are seen with increasing frequency as age advances and there are several important differences between young and old. Osteoarthritic changes in major weight bearing joints, such as hips, knees and spine are rarely significant in the young and almost universal in the old. Their assessment and management are different and will be discussed in more detail below. For example, the sudden onset of backache in an elderly person who has previously been symptom-free is almost always a sign of significant metabolic or neoplastic bone disease. Rheumatoid disease of small and medium sized joints is most frequently seen in younger people, but may sometimes occur for the first time in late life. Usually these joints, when affected in an older person, are the result of the late secondary osteoarthritic changes following old, burnt-out rheumatoid arthritis. Ligamentous and tendon inflammation in an old person may be associated with other diseases – especially strokes and osteoarthritis.

Bone disease of ageing is a general term to embrace osteoporotic and osteomalacic changes. Both are very common in the elderly and often co-existent. Their differentiation is important, but sometimes impossible and they will be discussed in detail elsewhere. Specific bone disease in the old includes Paget's disease of bone, which occurs in at least 1% of all those over 65 years with a steadily increasing incidence after that age. Secondary neoplastic disease in bone is also common in the elderly and may arise from the prostate in men, the breast in women, and from the lung, thyroid and gut in both.

Metabolic disease such as maturity-onset diabetes or gout is frequently seen in the elderly. Quite often it is associated with inappropriate treatment, especially with diuretic drugs. Late-onset diabetes mellitus is associated with excessive body weight and is complicated by a high incidence of micro-vascular disease, particularly affecting the eye and the autonomic nervous system as well as the peripheral circulation of the legs. Good control of the blood sugar levels does not seem to improve the complications that are associated with these changes.

Dementia has been estimated to be as high as 20% in the population over 80 years, although recent studies have suggested that this figure is probably grossly exaggerated. Nevertheless, impairment of higher mental functions appears to be a common feature of ageing, as in the 'senile' type of dementia, and may be associated with generalized vascular disease in 'arteriosclerotic' dementia. From whatever cause, dementia imposes great problems on the patients' family and friends as well as on the primary health care team. The natural tendency of the elderly to become increasingly socially isolated by bereavement, deterioration of hearing and visual acuity and diminished physical mobility is greatly exaggerated by the dementing process. A vicious circle of increasingly anti-social behaviour may make the elderly person unacceptable to live with in his normal environment.

Depressive disease is very common in the elderly, partly because of the social and physical deterioration that contributes to the problems of dementia. It may also be difficult to differentiate depressive disease from dementia, or it may indeed co-exist with it. Endogenous depression is also frequently seen in the elderly and may be difficult to treat. The incidence of successful suicide in the elderly is much higher than in the young.

SPECIAL FACTORS IN THE MANAGEMENT OF DISEASE IN THE ELDERLY

There are several important ways in which the care of the elderly differs from that of younger people:

Superimposed upon disease in the elderly are the complications of ageing changes. Indeed, ageing changes may themselves give rise to symptoms which bring the patient into contact with the general practitioner.

Disease in the old is rarely isolated and usually there are at least two identifiable diseases in the same patient. The coexistence of more than one disease, and the associated ageing changes that are inevitable in the elderly patient, modify the symptomatology of a single disease and introduce complications in any therapeutic moves that are made.

An understanding of the normal ageing processes that can be expected in an elderly person is essential, both in the assessment of the symptomatology and in the method of management.

AGEING CHANGES

Ageing changes occur in all body systems, but the most important ones as far as management of the sick elderly person is concerned are those in the heart and circulatory system, the brain, the kidney and the gut.

Cardiovascular system

Ageing changes in the *heart* affect the muscle, the conducting tissue and the valves. Even in the absence of coronary artery disease there is some muscle loss and fibrosis. In addition ageing brings about the development of senile cardiac amyloidisis. The net result of these changes is that there is a reduction in the resting cardiac output by as much as 30% at the age of 75 compared with that in a 30-year-old.

The *heart valves* may become calcified with age, and this is most marked in the aortic valve. The mitral valve may be affected by mucoid degeneration as well. Sclerosis of the aortic valve usually leads to loss of pliability and thus a minor degree of regurgitation is more likely than stenotic obstruction. The degeneration in the mitral valve produces some incompetence, and if it also affects the papillary muscle gives rise to the characteristic click and late systolic murmur that is heard when the posterior cusp prolapses. The functional result of these valve changes is not usually severe, and the main importance is the old person's susceptibility to infective endocarditis.

The most important ageing changes in the heart are those affecting the *conducting system*. The sino-atrial node is gradually replaced by fibrosis, leading to failing dominance of the cardiac pacemaker. The most frequent result of this is the development of atrial fibrillation, which occurs in at least 12% of all those over the age of 70 years. Other features of the sick sinus syndrome include severe sinus bradycardia, alternating periods of bradycardia and tachycardia (bradycardia-tachycardia syndrome) and sino-atrial block. The atrio-ventricular node and the His bundles also become fibrotic with age and lead to an increasingly high incidence of bundle branch block and complete heart block.

Atheromatous deposition in all the *main arteries* has usually reached its maximum by the sixth decade. These changes are associated both with vessel narrowing and a loss of elasticity. Thus arterial atheroma contributes both to the progressive rise of the systolic blood pressure and widening pulse pressure with age as well as to a reduction in regional blood flow.

Kidneys

Blood flow to the kidneys falls to about one half of the early adult flow by 85 years of age. Glomerular filtration falls by an equivalent amount. Interstitial fibrosis and fibrotic changes in the glomeruli occur even in the absence of hypertension. It has been estimated that there is a reduction in the number of functioning nephrons of 50% by the eighth decade. The functional changes in the kidney are extremely important with regard to the old person's ability to handle a great variety of drugs. Renal functional impairment with age is almost universal and may well not be demonstrated by any rise in the blood levels of urea or creatinine.

Brain

Ageing changes in the brain are probably not directly related to the minor fall in cerebral blood flow with age. There is a progressive loss of cerebral substance which may start in early adulthood. Cerebral atrophy may lead to dementia – the new epidemic of the late twentieth century.

Gut

The main ageing problems in the gut are the result of both small vessel and nerve degeneration. Ischaemia of the bowel may reduce adsorption and, if extreme, both small and large bowel necrosis. Malabsorptive states affect drug metabolism rather more than they do vital nutrients. Neurological problems with gut largely affect the lower bowel and contribute to the symptom of constipation, which is such a problem in many old people. The high incidence of diverticulosis is more a result of decades of poor diet low in roughage than a true degenerative disorder.

THE CAUSES AND PREVENTION OF DISABILITY AND DISEASE

Unfortunately our present knowledge has demonstrated very few factors that can be modified in younger life in order to slow down the inexorable decay of body structures.

Clearly the *control of hypertension* in young and middle aged persons will prevent the acceleration of atherosclerosis, and has been shown to reduce the incidence of stroke disease and possibly the incidence of myocardial infarction.

Similarly *modification of dietary habits* can be shown to lower the incidence of many diseases, such as coronary heart disease, strokes and diverticulosis, by the intake of high levels of roughage and a small intake of cholesterol and sugars.

The progress of *cerebral degeneration* may be accelerated by chronically high levels of intake of poisons, such as alcohol. Uncontrolled hypertension will also increase the incidence of ischaemic vascular disease of the brain. However, as yet there is no known cause of the development of senile dementia, despite the vigorous efforts of research workers over many years.

The *prevention of osteoporosis* is one of the areas where there is scope for considerable improvement. Bone loss with ageing occurs in both sexes but is most marked in women after the menopause. Clinical osteoporosis occurs when the bone mass reduces below a critical level, and is thus much more common in postmenopausal women with a small adult bone mass.

Slowing of the normal bone loss with ageing can be achieved by the administration of cyclical oestrogens, although one has to balance the proven benefit of this form of therapy with the problem of continued uterine bleeding and the possible cardiovascular problems that may occur. Calcium administration is of very dubious value since most people in the United Kingdom take an adequate amount of calcium in their diet.

The most practicable preventive for the development of osteoporosis is continued physical activity, since immobility is a powerful cause of localised osteoporosis, especially of the spine and femur.

Prevention of psychiatric disease in the elderly is another area that requires attention. Depression, with a very real risk of suicide, is often caused by social and intellectual isolation. Promotion of the continued cohesion of the family unit and social integration may do much to prevent psychological illness in old people. We need a radical revision in our current practices of 'parking' old people in residential homes when they become a 'social problem' and an increase in the provision of support services in the community so that they can spend more of their later years in their own homes. The technological advance in communication aids is just one such factor that needs to be employed more widely.

ATTITUDES TO MANAGEMENT

This is an area which requires great skill from the general practitioner. Old people respond very satisfactorily to treatment of the vast majority of diseases. Accurate diagnosis and assessment of their problems are essential, and frequently not at all easy.

With modern physical and chemical therapy many illnesses, previously thought to be incurable or just due to old age, can be alleviated or even cured. The single feature that distinguishes treatment of disease in the old person, as compared to the young, is that it takes more time to take effect. The outlook for survivors of acute stroke disease should be good. To achieve a good result, however, it is necessary to involve a large number of services and different disciplines at a very early stage of the illness.

It is very important to take a positive approach in treating the elderly, and treatment of all illnesses must be started early before other systems begin to break down. The importance of early treatment and mobilization is well exemplified in the case of an acute illness such as bronchopneumonia or myocardial infarction. Bed rest should be kept to a minimum of 24 hours, except in exceptional circumstances, since otherwise the elderly will rapidly lose their postural reflexes and muscle tone. If this happens it may take weeks or months to attain the previous level of independence.

PRINCIPLES OF PRESCRIBING

Correct drug treatment in the elderly is absolutely critical for many reasons. Two whole books have recently been published on this subject and the notes here can only be regarded as a summary.

Drug *compliance* is vital for therapeutic success. The minimum number of drugs to be taken in a day should be prescribed in order to avoid confusion over pills. If possible once a day drugs having a long action should be used.

The *unwanted effects* of individual drugs should be thoroughly understood as well as drug interaction, since many old people are taking several different agents at any one time.

The actual *packaging* of drugs is important, since those with arthritic hands may find great difficulty in opening bottles or measuring spoonfuls of liquid medicines.

Careful *explanation* should be given to the patient, and if possible the relatives, about why the drug is being prescribed, how to take it and what unwanted effects may occur. It is usually a good idea to write out details of treatment as old people may forget or become confused about treatment; this is especially important in the case of a reducing course of steroids.

A *drug cooperation card* is very useful and is already used by many general practitioners, but these cards are useless unless they are kept up to date and always used by both patient and doctor.

Drug metabolism may be markedly affected by the ageing process, and this applies mostly to drugs excreted by the kidney. However there are many groups of drugs that need to be given in the same dosage as in younger adults; these include antibiotics, steroids, most analgesics and anti-inflammatory agents as well as diurectics.

The most important renally excreted drug that causes severe toxic problems is *digoxin*. Most old people, even with normal levels of blood urea, are adequately treated with doses of 0.0625–0.125 mg daily. For those with blood urea levels two to three times the upper limit of normal the dosage may be as low as 0.0625 mg three times a week.

Many of the *beta-adrenergic block agents* are excreted by the kidney and the dosage should always be started at a low level and increased slowly if necessary.

Drug interactions and unwanted effects of individual drugs are a greater problem in the old than the young. The constipating effect of many analgesics, simple antacids, and anti-arrhythmic drugs, such as disopyramide, may cause crippling symptoms in the old. The atropinic effects of many agents may precipitate glaucoma or severe prostatism. Diuretic agents may light up a diabetic state or severely exacerbate existing diabetes as well as upsetting the potassium status of the old.

Perhaps the biggest practical problem in prescribing for the elderly is *multiple prescribing* with long lists of medications that they may be taking. This not only enhances the risk of drug interaction but also reduces the likelihood of drug compliance. It is important also to remove old and unfinished courses of tablets from the home and to review each patient's drug regimen at frequent intervals. If the patient is attending the surgery it is worth encouraging them to bring all their drugs with them to ensure that they understand exactly what pills they are taking and when they should take them.

THE NATURE OF SOME COMMON DISEASES

Old age sees a *continuation of the major diseases of middle age*, such as the vascular diseases of the heart, circulation and the brain, the whole range of neoplastic diseases and the chronic diseases such as rheumatoid arthritis and chronic lung disease.

In addition there are some illnesses that are virtually *peculiar to old age*, such as polymalgia rheumatica, myeloma, Paget's disease of bone, prostatism and osteoporosis.

Superimposed upon these problems are the *effects of ageing changes in most body systems*, which modify the symptomatology, the individual's ability to respond to disease, the complications of management and, not least, the physician's attitude to old age itself.

It will quickly be appreciated that one is not dealing with a single disease entity, but usually a *combination of at least two coincidental illnesses and a number of other factors* related to ageing changes. In view of this the second section of this book will deal with problem symptomatology and investigate the differential diagnosis, bearing in mind that it is not necessary to try and find one single cause for any particular problem. This represents a major deviation from attitudes which may be appropriate in the medicine of younger patients. Perhaps more than in any other area of general medicine one really has to consider the whole patient both from a medical and social point of view. The results from careful assessment and skilful treatment can be very rewarding, but, as always, one's attitude should be to maintain and improve the quality of life rather than merely to attempt to prolong it. In large measure we now have the ability to do this, and if this work can provide some helpful suggestions then our efforts will have been amply rewarded.

ORGANIZATION OF CARE FOR THE ELDERLY

The challenges faced by the general practitioner in the provision of care for the elderly are considerable. In addition to the requisite knowledge of normal ageing and the different presentations and courses of disease in the elderly, the general practitioner must also be aware of the services available in the community and how to mobilize these services for the benefit of individual patients and their families. He must also know how to organize his practice so that the special needs of the elderly are met. After all, in the National Health Service he is paid an additional fee as a recognition of the extra workload produced by this group of patients. He must be aware of the limitations of the traditional symptom–presentation model of medical care for the elderly but he must also guard against falling into the trap of routine or 'chronic' visiting, which may rapidly become devoid of any medical content at all and represent an uneconomic use of limited resources. Total prevention of disease is rarely possible, but onset may be delayed and disability minimized if problems are picked up early and simple preventive precautions are taken. Painful feet can be more of a handicap than mild cardiac failure, and the resultant lack of mobility and social contact may lead to depression and suicide. Similarly, a fall on a loose mat may lead to a fractured femur, subsequent pneumonia and death. Thus there is a strong case for a preventive approach to the elderly, especially those over 75 years old or living alone and housebound as these are the categories most likely to be at risk.

At present about 15% of the population are over 65 years of age, perhaps 1500 in a typical group practice serving 10 000 patients. Between 65 and 75, women outnumber men by about two to one, after 75 the ratio is nearer three to one. The elderly population will increase to a peak of nearly 20% by the end of the present century, when the number over 75 years will almost equal those between 65 years and 75 years. Unfortunately, there is no evidence that all those extra people who live to 75 years and beyond will be more healthy than their counterparts today.

Beyond 80 years of age, many people cease to be able to lead an independent existence. Those unable to live at home without assistance increase

11

from 12% between 65-69 years to over 80% at 85 years. Nevertheless, one in four of those aged 85 years or more live on their own before death. Ninety five per cent of pensioners live at home and are cared for by their general practitioners and 40% of all general practitioner's consultations are with the elderly already. Thus by the year 2000 more than one half of the general practitioner's workload will be concerned with the care of the elderly. The real possibility exists that the primary care services will be overwhelmed by the increased workload unless steps are taken to rationalize the services provided and organize the practice to meet the needs. Every practice should know who their elderly patients are, where they live and what their unmet needs and problems are. This implies a need for an accurate age-sex register, and an up-to-date list of the names and addresses of all people over 65 years, with a note of whether or not they are attending surgery or visited regularly by the doctor, nurse or health visitor, and a special note of those at risk because they live alone, have recently been bereaved or are without social support. Patients who are not known to the team, especially those over 75 years, may be visited by a doctor or nurse in order to ascertain unmet needs. The practice nurse or health visitor can readily assess the patient at home and involve the doctor if required. A simple check list of possible problems should include such questions as:

Can the patient get out and about?
Can they get around the house?
Can they wash and dress themselves?
Can they obtain and cook their food?
Can they keep warm?
Have they got enough money?
Can they keep clean?
Are they safe?
Can they communicate with other people?
Are they happy?
Have they got any necessary medicines? If so, do they know what they are for and how to take them?

It is usually quite readily apparent from such an assessment whether the patient requires further investigation by the doctor, regular surveillance by a nurse or, wherever possible, to be left alone to get on with their life. Some doctors feel that regular screening examinations are necessary but these are expensive and time-consuming, and often not appreciated by the patients. It seems more likely that concentration by the doctor on high risk groups will be most cost-effective, provided that team members are constantly on the lookout for insidious conditions such as hypothyroidism and anaemia which are quite common in the elderly.

Thus, by organizing his practice efficiently, the general practitioner can control his workload, rationalize the services provided and improve the quality of care of all his elderly patients, rather than just those who present themselves to him.

Section 2

Symptoms and their Differential Diagnosis

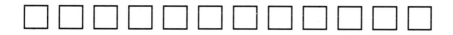

In this section symptom complexes that are frequently seen in general practice are identified. The significance of these symptoms is discussed, and the diseases that may be associated with them are outlined. More detailed discussion of most of these diseases, together with their management, will be found in the third section of this book.

PALPITATIONS

Palpitations are common at all ages but may be a major problem to the old. Patients may recognize very many different forms of palpitations. These may vary from a sensation of accentuated beating of the heart, a pounding in the chest and neck, a fluttering in the chest or an obvious irregularity of the heart action. Time in the surgery will be well spent in determining exactly what the patient means by palpitations, as the causes can usually be accurately determined by careful history-taking. In particular, associated symptoms such as breathlessness and giddiness will help to differentiate between anxiety and a significant cardiac dysrhythmia.

Common causes

Anxiety
Cardiac dysrhythmias
Thyrotoxicosis
Systolic hypertension (arteriosclerosis).

Differential diagnosis

Relatively slow and regular pounding of the heart, chest wall, neck or head is likely to be associated with either anxiety or systolic hypertension. Patients who can accurately give this description, especially when it is not associated with dyspnoea or light-headedness, are unlikely to be suffering significant cardiac dysrhythmias. Supporting findings on clinical examination, such as obvious agitation, difficulty in getting off to sleep, cold sweaty hands and a resting heart rate of 90–120 beats per minute point strongly to anxiety as a cause. Many of these elderly patients may have concern about their physical health, family problems or worries about their financial or social situation.

Clinical findings such as thickened peripheral arteries with systolic hypertension and a wide pulse pressure may elucidate another group of patients with harmless symptoms.

Irregular beating of the heart, especially when it is associated with other symptoms such as breathlessness, chest pain or light-headedness almost always points to a serious cardiac dysrhythmia. The most common of these is paroxysmal atrial fibrillation. During the paroxysms the heart rate is usually very fast (120–200 per minute). Although the history may be clear, the accurate demonstration of a cardiac dysrhythmia may be difficult, since the paroxysms are often short-lived and are rarely present when the doctor is in attendance. Electrocardiographic proof is therefore rare, and accurate documentation can usually only be provided by continuous ambulatory monitoring of the heart rhythm by dynamic electrocardiographic monitoring (DCG).

BREATHLESSNESS

Dyspnoea is such a common symptom in the elderly that it is often regarded by patients as being a normal accompaniment of ageing. Certainly pulmonary and cardiac functions decrease with age and exertional dyspnoea may be an unremarkable finding. Assessment of this symptom demands expert clinical judgement.

Common causes

Cardiac failure
Chest infections
Infiltrative pulmonary disease
Cardiac dysrhythmias

16

Emphysema
Pneumothorax
Anaemia.

Assessment

Dyspnoea may only occur on exertion. The doctor must then assess whether the level of exertion that produces breathlessness is unreasonable or not. Many old people have an unrealistic expectation of performance. It is probably unreasonable for an eighty-year-old person who is not normally active to be able to hurry up stairs or to run for a bus, for example. On the other hand a person of similar age, who has always been active should reasonably expect to be able to walk a mile without discomfort. Assessment of dyspnoea must take into account the general fitness and activity level of the individual, and in this situation the general practitioner is usually in a unique position to make this judgement. Any sudden diminution of exercise tolerance points to significant disease. Other factors that should be taken into account in assessment of exertional dyspnoea are locomotor problems such as osteoarthritis of the major joints and parkinsonism, which demand the production of increased muscular energy in order to overcome the musculoskeletal problem.

Dyspnoea at rest or during resting in bed at night is always pathological and indicative of serious pulmonary or cardiac disease. These symptoms are often associated with other findings, such as oedema of the ankles, cough and sputum production or palpitations.

Differential diagnosis

If exertional dyspnoea is judged to be pathological it may be caused by any of the conditions listed above. Pulmonary causes are usually associated with cough and sputum production and, sometimes, wheezing. Cardiac causes of exertional dyspnoea are usually associated with ankle oedema or chest pain and sometimes palpitations. Many of the patients with heart disease will also have orthopnoea and paroxysmal nocturnal dyspnoea. Very often a mixed picture of both pulmonary and cardiac disease will be seen.

A rapidly changing picture of exertional dyspnoea associated with fever and purulent sputum clearly points to an infective cause in the lungs, but a more gradually developing situation may indicate infiltrative lung disease, either from fibrosis due to dust diseases or rheumatoid arthritis, or neoplastic infiltration from primary lung cancer or secondary spread to the lungs from tumours in other sites.

Dyspnoea at rest is always pathological and is indicative of severe pulmonary disease, such as infection, emphysema and infiltrative disease, and may be associated with unilateral pleural effusion or pneumothorax. Other physical signs, such as polycythaemia, finger clubbing or rheumatoid changes in the hands may help to interpret the lung disease. Cardiac causes of dyspnoea at rest are easier to recognize, since they are often associated with ankle oedema, chest pain, palpitations or orthopnoea.

Paroxysmal noctural dyspnoea (PND) is almost always cardiac in origin. The commonest cause in the elderly is paroxysmal atrial fibrillation with a rapid ventricular rate producing left ventricular failure. Myocardial infarction, occasionally silent, may produce a similar picture. Less often seen nowadays as a cause of PND are valvular lesions of rheumatic origin, but senile valvular disease, especially with cusp rupture or prolapse is increasingly being recognized. In the elderly hypertensive heart disease very rarely causes left ventricular failure.

COUGH

Cough is a symptom that brings patients of all ages to their general practitioner. In the elderly the first question to ask is whether it is dry or productive. It is also necessary to ascertain whether it is associated with pain, fever or dyspnoea.

Common causes

Dry	*Productive*
Tracheitis	Post-nasal drip
Bronchial tumours	Chronic bronchitis
Infiltrative lung disease	Chest infections
	Bronchial tumours

Differential diagnosis

Dry cough is most commonly due to viral tracheitis and the patient usually has other manifestations, such as myalgia and upper respiratory symptoms. Bronchial tumours and infiltrative lung disease may present with dry cough but there are usually other symptoms such as anorexia and weight loss. Cough due to hysteria is sometimes seen in the elderly and is probably the only feature of true hysteria seen in this age group; but this diagnosis can only be made after exhaustive investigation and exclusion of other conditions.

Productive cough is frequently seen in the old and is most usually due to chronic bronchitis. The diagnosis is generally easy, since the history is long and most of these patients have smoked heavily and often continue to do so. Changing patterns of sputum colour and quantity usually indicate exacerbations of acute infection. Associated weight loss and anorexia should raise the possibility of the development of bronchial carcinoma, and these patients may also have haemoptysis. The chronic expectoration of purulent sputum, especially associated with finger clubbing indicates bronchiectasis. Any deterioration in a previously stable situation in these patients should alert the doctor to the possibility of the development of a bronchial neoplasm, and is an indication to perform a chest X-ray. Wheezing may frequently develop in the patients with chronic bronchitis and is almost always due to superadded infection, but on occasion may herald the development of heart failure or a bronchial tumour.

SWOLLEN LEGS

Ankle oedema is frequently seen in the elderly and is often a pointer to significant underlying disease.

Common causes

Gravitational
Congestive cardiac failure
Hypoproteinaemia
Venous or lymphatic obstruction.

Differential diagnosis

The commonest cause of ankle swelling is gravitational oedema, sometimes associated with venous varicosity. Dependent oedema may occur in anyone if the normal muscle pump in the legs is not activated, as any aeroplane traveller will know. The elderly often spend a great deal of time sitting in chairs and there are countless thousands of people taking diuretic agents inappropriately for this condition. The role of the general practitioner in elucidating this condition is unique, since he is likely to be the only doctor to have the chance to see the patient at home. In the surgery or in hospital clinics the history of physical inactivity is so often denied by the patient. Many of these patients also have some degree of leg vein varicosity which will exacerbate the situation.

Hypoproteinaemia is not uncommon in the elderly, usually due to chronic malnutrition but sometimes associated with renal or hepatic disease. There are often other manifestations of these other conditions, such as anaemia or weight loss.

Cardiac failure is a sign of disease and not a cause. Elderly patients with chronic ankle oedema deserve full clinical examination of the heart to exclude ischaemic or valvular disease. Their inactivity is exaggerated by the associated weakness and dyspnoea on exertion.

Leg oedema is usully bilateral, but if it is unilateral care must be taken to determine an obstructive cause in either the venous or lymphatic drainage.

'GOING OFF HIS FEET' SYNDROME

This syndrome is used to describe a whole rag bag of conditions that produce immobility in the elderly, many of which may occur in harmony.

Common causes

Osteoarthritis
Rheumatoid arthritis
Gout and pseudogout
Cerebrovascular disease
Parkinsonian syndromes
Cervical spondylosis
Polymyalgia rheumatica
Osteomalacia
Visual deterioration
Postural hypotension
Disorders of balance
Depression.

Differential diagnosis

All of the above diseases are common in the elderly and several may co-exist in the same patient. The list is by no means exhaustive and within each heading there are many subgroups. The common denominator to all is significant disablement, failure to lead an independent existence and increasing demands on family, nursing and social services. The importance in clearly identifying the cause or causes of increasing immobility cannot be overstressed, since a great deal can be done to ameliorate and overcome the problems. Careful history-taking and clinical examination are essential.

Aggressive investigation and treatment is often indicated if the problems are to be overcome. A large section of this book is devoted to the identification and management of these conditions.

FITS, FAINTS AND FALLS

These symptoms are very frequently found in the elderly and may often be associated with the 'gone off his feet' syndrome.

Common causes

Epilepsy
Postural hypotension
Cardiac arrhythmias
Extracranial artery disease
Vaso-vagal attacks
Locomotor instability.

Differential diagnosis

Fits in the elderly are usually due to epileptic seizures and are nearly always due to cerebrovascular disease, intracranial tumours or cardiac arrhythmias. Even careful history-taking will rarely accurately identify the cause of a fit since the natural history of cerebrovascular disease and intracranial tumours may be so variable. The general guide that intracranial tumours produce slowly progressive symptoms, and cerebrovascular disease acutely presenting symptoms, is probably true but not accurate enough to exclude one or the other. Cardiac arrhythmias usually produce episodic symptoms of fits, but in all cases extensive investigation is required. This will include a full cardiovascular and neurological examination, chest X-ray, resting ECG and dynamic ambulatory ECG and, usually, a CT brain scan.

Symptoms of faintness and light-headedness are common and are generally due to reduced intracranial blood perfusion, although less clear symptoms may be caused by anxiety. Reduced blood flow to the brain is most commonly caused by a fall in the perfusion pressure as a result of *postural hypotension*. *Drugs* are a major cause of this problem, whether anti-hypertensive agents such as methyldopa or drugs of the vasodilator group, such as prazosin. Inappropriate treatment of measurable elevation of the blood pressure with any drug will cause the same effect, and emphasizes the importance of measuring the standing blood pressure before any treatment is started. Phenothiazine drugs, such as chlorpromazine also cause fall in systemic blood pressure. *Autonomic instability*, often associated with Type II diabetes, also affects the control of postural blood pressure and is an important cause of 'faint' spells.

Extracranial arterial disease, such as carotid artery stenosis and subclavian steal syndrome, is an important cause of faintness and may be associated with cervical spondylosis. It is important to include auscultation of the neck in the general examination to exclude carotid or subclavian bruits.

Faintness may be described by patients with vertigo due to *middle ear disease* and examination of the ear and vestibular apparatus should never be omitted.

Disturbances of cardiac rhythm, due either to paroxysmal tachycardias or bradycardia may produce profound reduction in intracranial perfusion, especially when associated with extracranial arterial disease. *Hypotensive states* may also occur in other cardiac conditions, especially myocardial infarction and left ventricular outflow tract obstruction.

Vaso-vagal attacks caused by hypersensitive carotid sinuses are not uncommon in the elderly and produce a profound bradycardia and fall in systemic blood pressure. The best described examples are micturition syncope on straining in men with prostatic disease and cough syncope in elderly bronchitics, but it may also occur whilst shaving due to pressure on the carotid sinus in susceptible subjects.

More severe examples of the causes of faintness mentioned above may lead to syncope and, on occasion, fits.

The great majority of falls in the elderly are *accidental*, caused by tripping over loose mats and wires. They are often associated with visual impairment, whether due to cataracts, retinopathy or hemianopia. A rare form of visual disturbance occurs in *progressive supra nuclear palsy* (Steele–Richardson syndrome) where there is paralysis of downward gaze. *Bifocal spectacle lenses* make descending stairs extremely hazardous and most people take a long time to adjust to them.

Falls are also increased in old people with locomotor instability, such as *strokes, Parkinson's disease* and *osteoarthritis* of the major leg joints.

Patients with the problems already described in faints are much more likely to fall than healthy old people.

ACHES AND PAINS

A very large amount of a general practitioner's time is taken up by elderly people complaining of aches and pains, often in the shoulders and spine. Accurate diagnosis is often difficult and as a result treatment is frequently symptomatic and inappropriate.

Common causes

Osteoarthritis of the spine
Osteoporosis and osteomalacia
Rheumatoid arthritis
Polymyalgia rheumatica
Secondary malignancy

These musculo-skeletal pains in the elderly are a very real source of misery and, often, significant disability. Examination of the spine may give some clues as to the diagnosis if, for instance, kyphosis, muscular spasm or diminished movements are noted. Nerve root pain must be looked for as its presence indicates urgent and active treatment. Proximal muscle weakness may indicate *osteomalacia* and gives rise to a characteristic waddling gait and difficulty in climbing stairs. Shoulder girdle pain, especially if there is tenderness and mild fever, is characteristic of *polymyalgia rheumatica*. Shoulder pain may also be caused by *cervical spondylosis* and it is important to differentiate a spinal cause of the pain from a more local cause such as rheumatic disease of the shoulder. Occasionally infection may be the cause of back pain and there is usually local tenderness and fever. *Secondary deposits* in the spine from a primary malignancy in the breast, prostate, kidney or lung should always be borne in mind, especially when the history of backache is short and the patient has had no previous trouble in this area.

The majority of these cases cannot be accurately diagnosed without X-rays of the neck or spine. In many people blood tests of bone chemistry are essential to exclude osteomalacia and metastatic bone disease. In polymyalgia rheumatica rapid acceleration of the ESR is almost always found.

CONSTIPATION AND DIARRHOEA

Disturbances of large bowel function are very common in the elderly and may pose difficult problems in management.

Common causes

Inadequate diet
Diverticulosis
Drugs
Large bowel cancer
Spurious diarrhoea
Infections of the lower gut

Differential diagnosis

Constipation in the elderly is so common that the majority of old people are chronic laxative takers. Probably because of the very long standing habit of eating low roughage foods in Western society, *diverticulosis* is almost universal in the present elderly population. This phenomenon together with physical inactivity and autonomic denervation of the large bowel with ageing leads to chronic constipation. Changing bowel habit, however, is a warning sign that *large bowel cancer* is present. This may be associated with bleeding and requires full endoscopic and barium enema examination.

Many drugs can cause constipation, including antacids, tranquillisers and analgesics.

Impaction of faeces may occur in the rectum and is associated with massive dilatation of the rectum and often with very lax abdominal wall musculature. Many of these patients have faecal soiling or incontinence. *Myxoedema and depression* are also important causes of constipation. Impaction of faeces higher up in the colon is not uncommon and may lead to spurious diarrhoea.

Diarrhoea may be associated with large bowel neoplasms but is most frequently due to intestinal infections, to which the elderly are highly susceptible. Thus stool examination for both occult blood and micro-organisms is mandatory in cases of diarrhoea.

FAILING EYESIGHT AND HEARING

Failing eyesight and hearing are an inevitable accompaniment of ageing, but there are many conditions which are potentially correctable. Loss of visual acuity not only increases the likelihood of falls but reduces the quality of life by making reading and watching television much more difficult. Hearing loss also promotes social isolation and increases the general frustrations of ageing.

Common causes

Loss of visual acuity

Loss of accommodation
Cataract
Macular degeneration
Glaucoma

Retinal artery occlusion
Field defect loss

Hearing loss

Presbyacusis
Meniere's disease
Wax

Differential diagnosis

Progressive lens inelasticity with age is inevitable and presents with increasing blurring of near vision. *Open angle glaucoma* is also of insidious onset and causes blurring of vision and there is usually a field defect when the patient presents to the doctor. *Angle-closure glaucoma* presents much more acutely and is associated with pain.

Cataract formation occurs in about 5% of the elderly population, but is much more common in diabetics.

Macular degeneration is both common and progressive and is caused by new vessel formation in the macular area. In advanced cases the pigmentary stippling is very marked and there are surrounding white areas of choridal atrophy.

Visual field defects are common after *hemiplegia* and may be very disabling. Sudden loss of vision in one eye is usually a result of *temporal arteritis*, but may be due to *micro-emboli* from the heart or carotid arteries. Retinal vein occlusion is rare, but may occur in macroglobulinaemia or polycythaemia. Retinal detachment is another cause of sudden loss of vision.

Presbyacusis implies the progressive loss of high tone hearing that is an inevitable accompaniment of ageing. This leads to difficulties in distinguishing tones of different frequencies, the direction of sound and the time relationship of sound. Occasionally speech may be impaired. Confirmation of the diagnosis is made by audiometry.

Meniere's syndrome consists of the triad of vertigo, deafness and tinnitus, although they do not all start at the same time. The deafness tends to be progressive and the vertigo paroxysmal. There may also be nausea and vomiting. The vertigo can be tested by caloric tests.

INCONTINENCE

Urinary and faecal incontinence probably cause more embarrassment and distress to patients and their carers than any other symptom. They also account for a significant number of long term hospital admissions as they are socially unacceptable.

Common causes

Urinary incontinence	*Faecal incontinence*
Faecal impaction	Faecal impaction
Immobility	Purgative abuse
Drugs	Diarrhoea
Urinary tract infection	Neurogenic
Pelvic floor muscle weakness	
Senile vaginitis	
Prostatism	
Neurogenic	

Differential diagnosis

Many cases of both urinary and faecal incontinence are relatively easily and accurately diagnosed provided a careful history is taken and a proper pelvic examination performed. The most difficult cases are those who have a *neurogenic* cause for their urinary incontinence. Because this is such an important area of management of the elderly and is related to the patho-physiological consequences of bladder function, a whole section on this will be found later in the book.

CONFUSION

Confusion in elderly patients will present the general practitioner with some of his most difficult problems. It is quite frequently a symptom that is reversible if diagnosed and treated in time and, therefore, it is important to take an aggressive approach to the problem.

Common causes

Toxic state
Dementia: arteriosclerotic/senile
Drug induced
Pre-senile dementia
Cerebro-vascular insufficiency
Depression

Psychosis
Myxoedema.

Differential diagnosis

By definition dementia in any form is irreversible. It is, therefore, important to exclude the other causes of confusion which are usually correctable.

Depression is common in the elderly and may present with some of the features of dementia, such as apathy, confusion, memory loss and neglect. The two conditions may co-exist. In depression the memory loss tends to be patchy and the illness is generally more acute and less progressive than in dementia. If in doubt, a therapeutic trial of anti-depressant treatment is worthwhile.

Toxic confusional states may be due to acute or chronic infections, usually of the chest or urinary tract. Biochemical disturbances such as raised blood sugar or urea levels or low serum sodium and sugar levels may produce a similar picture. Toxic confusional states are usually acute in onset and improve fairly rapidly on treatment.

Drug-induced confusional states may be related to the biochemical disturbances mentioned above or be a direct reaction to the drug, such as occurs in some analgesics, tranquillisers and hypnotics. Long acting hypnotics, such as the barbiturate group and nitrazepam, should not be used in the elderly. Some drugs such as L-dopa may cause confusion as a result of lowering the systemic blood pressure. In all these cases a direct causal response to the drug is easily obtained from the history.

Cerebro-vascular insufficiency may cause confusion that is episodic and usually related to hypotensive states. Extracranial artery stenosis is usually detectable by finding bruits in the neck. Multiple small emboli from either a stenosed carotid artery or from the heart may produce a similar picture.

Psychotic states, such as paraphrenia, may produce confusion and have some of the features of dementia, but there is no memory impairment and the intellect is preserved.

Myxoedema is found in about 2% of all people over 65 years who are admitted to hospital and is often difficult to diagnose in patients who are seen frequently. The confusional state (myxoedema madness) is not always reversible even with adequate thyroid replacement. Myxoedema has a very insidious onset. In addition to the characteristic facies, weight gain, physical and mental slowing, constipation and hoarse voice, these patients may present with the carpal tunnel syndrome or hypothermia. At the bedside the simplest test is to elicit the slow relaxation phase of the tendon jerks, particularly of the ankle.

Folic acid and *Vitamin B$_{12}$ deficiency* states may also produce confusion and the latter may be associated with myxoedema. *Dementia* may be produced by these conditions if they are not treated swiftly. The commoner causes of dementia are the senile (primary neuronal) and arterio-sclerotic types. Some old people with pre-senile dementia survive into old age. This condition is rare and caused by such conditions as Alzheimer's and Pick's disease as well as Huntington's chorea. All dementias are slowly progressive and are characterized by loss of memory for recent events, confusion, socially unacceptable behaviour disorders, impairment of the intellect and disintegration of the personality. In the later stages physical deterioration occurs.

MISERY, APATHY AND SLEEP PROBLEMS

These symptoms are frequently seen by the general practitioner on his home visits. Patients with these problems may well not present to the surgery unless they are brought by a relative. Many old people accept misery and apathy as a normal accompaniment of getting old. It is not always generally realized that these symptoms are often the features of significant and reversible disease.

Common causes

Depression
Anxiety state
Social deprivation
Myxoedema
Diogenes syndrome.

Differential diagnosis

Depression has been mentioned above but is the most important cause of these symptoms. The disturbance of sleep pattern is usually characterized by early morning waking. *Anxiety states* may occur alone or be associated with depression. Hyperthyroidism must be excluded by eliciting the inevitable weight loss and either paroxysmal or established atrial fibrillation. In contrast to patients with anxiety, the palms of the hands are dry and warm. In the elderly *hyperthyroidism* may be 'masked' and the features that are seen in younger patients with Graves' disease, such as tremor, thyroid enlargement with bruits and lid lag, are absent.

Social deprivation in some elderly persons is found even in wealthy societies. This may be a primary cause of apathy and misery or be second-ary to disease such as dementia and depression.

The *Diogenes syndrome* is a bizarre condition, examples of which can be found in the patients of every general practitioner. The patients withdraw from society and refuse to accept help. They live in squalor and their houses can easily be recognized by the peeling and filthy paintwork and broken windows in an otherwise smart street. These patients are almost always of high intelligence and, before their retirement or bereavement, were of good social standing and had jobs in the professions. They are rarely short of money and do not suffer any recognizable psychiatric disorder. They also usually collect rubbish (syllogomania) which may be amassed to such a degree that there is little room in the house for habitation. Most of these cases present with an acute medical or surgical condition requiring admis-sion to hospital and these are associated with a very high mortality rate.

COLLAPSE

From time to time all general practitioners will be called to an old person who has collapsed. Although the emergency treatment will usually involve calling an ambulance to take the patient to hospital, there are certain conditions that should be recognized since they require treatment in the home or street.

Common causes

Hypoglycaemia
Myocardial infarction
Cardiac arrhythmia
Cerebrovascular accident
Hypothermia
Poisoning
Epilepsy.

Differential diagnosis

The diagnosis of *hypoglycaemia* is usually easy if the patient is either on insulin or oral hypoglycaemic drugs such as glibenclamide or chlorpropam-ide. The patient is cold and sweaty and responds rapidly to intravenous glucose or glucagon. These drugs should be in every medical bag as should blood glucose testing strips (Dextrostix). Some patients with hyperglycae-mia may be found in a state of collapse and these patients may not be previously known diabetics. They are dry and overbreathing. Some elderly patients on phenformin may have lactic acidosis or non-keto-acidotic coma, although in the latter condition the onset of coma occurs at a very late stage of the illness and is associated with very high blood sugars.

Cardiac arrhythmias may occur after an *acute myocardial infarction* or present as collapse without infarction. These are usually severe bradycardic states, either due to high grade atrio-ventricular block, profound sinus bradycardia or sinus arrest. The tachycardias that cause collapse are usually ventricular flutter or fibrillation, but occasionally atrial flutter or fibrillation without significant atrio-ventricular block may be associated with such a rapid heart rate that it cannot adequately support cerebral perfusion. The correct diagnosis can usually only be made by examining the ECG, but this is important for the long-term management should the patient survive the acute episode.

Cerebrovascular accidents are usually easy to diagnose because of the obvious paralysis, abnormal reflexes and extensor plantar responses. However, the reticular formation is responsible for alertness and relatively small and discrete lesions of the brain stem may disrupt the reticular formation and produce coma without long tract signs. On the other hand vascular lesions of the cortex have to be very extensive to produce coma.

Coma may also occur from large structural lesions in the posterior fossa, for example *abscesses, tumours or haematomas in the cerebellum,* and these produce coma by brain stem compression. Large unilateral cortical lesions may produce 'mass effect' and cause herniation of parts of the temporal lobe through the tentorium with secondary distortion of the brain stem.

Examination of the eyes will help elucidate these lesions. Large unreactive pupils suggest extensive brain stem abnormality. A unilateral large pupil indicates a third nerve lesion and suggests tentorial herniation. Bilateral pin point pupils are caused either by a pontine lesion or may be due to opiates. A positive 'doll's head' manoeuvre, where a positive response is movement of the eyes to the corners of the orbit when the head is rotated to each side, is helpful in excluding a brain stem lesion. In *drug-induced coma* or in extensive *cerebral cortical lesions* there is depression of the reflex eye movements but intact pupillary reflexes.

Epilepsy may be idiopathic in previously diagnosed epileptics, or caused as a result of a cerebrovascular accident, cerebral tumours or due to alcoholic excess.

Poisoning, as a result of self-administration of drugs, or, occasionally, accidental overdosage, can usually be diagnosed by finding empty bottles of tablets or suicide notes. These patients may be deeply comatose without focal neurological signs but with intact pupillary reflexes. They are often profoundly shocked. The mortality for suicide attempts in the elderly is very high. Other causes of intended or accidental poisoning with *chemicals*, such as weedkillers and insecticides, should be suspected, but coma is not usually present. Carbon monoxide poisoning in the elderly is now rare in Britain.

Hypothermia is defined as a core body temperature below 35°C. It is still a major problem in the elderly. Few of these patients suffer from myxoedema, although the facial appearance of a patient with hypothermia resembles myxoedematous facies. Hypothermia is usually secondary to other causes of collapse, especially strokes and fractures of the femur in people living alone who are not found for some time. Hypothermia may occur in the absence of a low ambient temperature if people are exposed for long enough, especially if they have been taking drugs of the phenothiazine group. These drugs paralyse the temperature regulating centre. Hypothermia has also been seen in immobile patients who live in unheated houses.

Section 3

Specific Disease Complexes

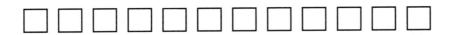

ABNORMALITIES OF BLOOD PRESSURE

What is hypertension in the elderly?

There are great difficulties in determining what does and what does not constitute hypertension in the elderly. It is possible to take almost any line of opinion and find some evidence to support it. However, we have taken a rather didactic line of approach in this section, not only for relative simplicity, but because we believe that there may be very serious implications in treating measured levels of blood pressure in the elderly over-enthusiastically.

For reasons that will be elaborated below, we define hypertension in the elderly as follows:

Aged	Men	Women
	Blood pressures greater than	
65-69 years	160/100	160/100
70-74 years	160/100	180/110
75 years or greater	Any level of blood pressure is acceptable	

These levels of blood pressure are based on the assumption that the measured blood pressure is taken on at least two separate occasions after resting for at least five minutes using an accurately placed and suitably sized cuff and a sphygmomanometer that is known to be accurate.

Aetiology

The blood pressure in the systemic circulation is governed by the *cardiac output* and the degree of the *peripheral resistance*. The cardiac output tends to fall with age, as a result of both ischaemic and degenerative disease of the myocardium. The latter may well be of paramount importance since it is only in recent years that the very high incidence of amyloid infiltration of the myocardium has been recognized in the elderly heart. Cardiac output may also be reduced in old people by the high incidence of degenerative valvular disease and by the occurrence of atrial fibrillation, which is found in at least 12% of otherwise healthy people over the age of 70 years.

Peripheral resistance in the elderly circulation may be markedly altered by degenerative changes in the sympathetic neurones that supply them. All these changes will be exaggerated in elderly diabetics. The importance of these changes in the peripheral circulation cannot be overemphasized since they not only lead to significant alterations of blood pressure with postural changes, but also lead to altered function of important target organs such as the kidney and brain. Unless these factors are properly assessed and understood, manipulation of the systemic blood pressure by drugs can lead to a dramatic deterioration in vital organ function and the exaggeration of postural hypotension.

Another factor that has to be considered in the elderly is the effect of atherosclerotic changes in the aorta and main arteries. The effect of an atherosclerotic aorta is to widen the pulse pressure since the rigid aorta fails to dampen the spikes of each ventricular systole. This situation leads to the phenomenon of so-called *'systolic hypertension'*. The dangers of treating apparently raised levels of systolic blood pressure when the diastolic pressure is normal or low can be very great, since all drugs tend to reduce both systolic and diastolic pressure and it is the latter that is responsible for adequate end-organ perfusion.

Atherosclerotic changes in the brachial artery may lead to erroneous measurement of the blood pressure by the indirect methods normally employed in clinical practice. It has long been established that the Korotkov phase V, when the sounds disappear, is the most accurate measurement of the diastolic pressure on indirect blood pressure measurement. Atherosclerotic changes in the brachial artery may make the assessment of the diastolic end-point impossible. Rhythm abnormalities of the heart, such as atrial fibrillation, may make accurate indirect assessment of the blood pressure by listening to the Korotkov phases extremely difficult.

Secondary hypertension as a result of renal disease or endocrine disorders, such as Conn's syndrome and phaechromocytoma, are so rare in the elderly that investigation is generally not indicated.

Clinical features

There are no specific clinical features of hypertension in the elderly. Headaches or epistaxes may occasionally occur, but a causal relationship is difficult to prove. Raised levels of blood pressure may be found at a casual examination, but again it must be stressed that a single blood pressure reading should never be regarded as an indication for treatment and should always be repeated on several occasions.

Complications

The evidence for a direct relationship between raised levels of blood pressure and cardiovascular and stroke disease remains the subject of much debate. It

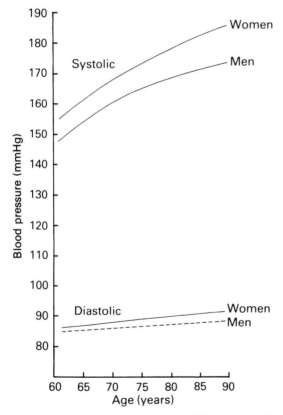

Figure 3.1   Rise in blood pressure with age in healthy subjects (from Martin (1981) *Problems in Geriatric Medicine*, p. 28 (Lancaster: MTP Press) with permission)

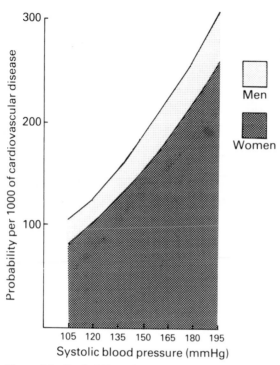

Figure 3.2 Probability of cardiovascular disease in 8 years in 70-year-olds according to systolic blood pressure (from Martin (1981) *Problems in Geriatric Medicine*, p. 30 (Lancaster: MTP Press) with permission)

has long been recognized that there is a progressive rise in the level of systolic blood pressure with increasing age (Figure 3.1). The most significant evidence for a relationship between raised levels of systolic blood pressure and an increase in the incidence of cardiovascular disease has come from the Framingham study in the United States (Figure 3.2). There is also some evidence from the United Kingdom that raised levels of diastolic blood pressure may be associated with an increase in the incidence of electrocardiographic abnormalities (Figure 3.3). Despite this, however, other work from London has shown that raised levels of blood pressure actually confer some benefit as far as survival in the 70 and over age group is concerned (Figure 3.4). Similarly, most of the well-controlled trials of treatment of hypertension in the elderly have failed to demonstrate any benefit in survival.

Very recently the European Working Party on High Blood Pressure in

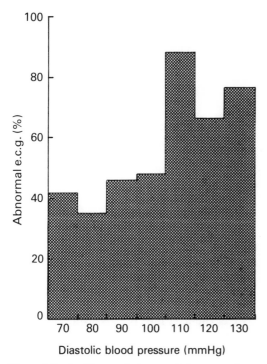

Figure 3.3 Incidence of abnormal electrocardiographs with diastolic blood pressure (from Martin (1981) *Problems in Geriatric Medicine*, p. 29 (Lancaster: MTP Press) with permission)

the Elderly (EWPHE) study has been reported. This study was set up in 1972 to ascertain the effects of drug treatment on the mortality and morbidity associated with raised blood pressure and also to assess adverse reactions of this treatment in elderly hypertensives. It has to be said from the outset that there are certain concerns about the validity of this study. Although this was a multi-centre study only 840 people were recruited over 12 years, which suggests that the sample may not have been representative of the elderly hypertensives in Europe at large. The admitting age to the study was 60 years or more and the blood pressure limits were 90–119 mm Hg diastolic which means that the results could have been unduly influenced by the treatment of the relatively young and very hypertensive group. Against this the treatment schedule could now be regarded as old-fashioned, since it consisted of a thiazide diuretic and methyldopa, whereas one would tend to use diuretics in smaller doses and beta-blockers at the present time. Despite these considerable reservations the EWPHE trial remains the best

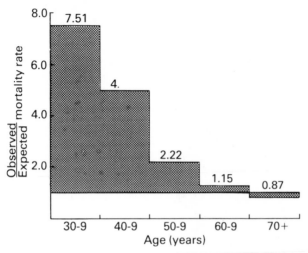

Figure 3.4 Observed/expected mortality at various ages (from Martin (1981) *Problems in Geriatric Medicine*, p. 30 (Lancaster: MTP Press) with permission)

that we have to date and this justifies the length of the discussion accorded to it.

The results of the EWPHE trial showed no significant effect on the overall mortality of treatment. Similarly there was no change in the mortality from cerebrovascular events. However, there was a significant reduction in the incidence of cardiovascular mortality (27%), cardiovascular events (38%) and non-fatal cerebrovascular events (50%). These results were achieved despite an increase in the amount of both biochemical and clinical gout and glucose intolerance.

Cardiac failure is a major complication of raised levels of blood pressure in younger people, and it is widely believed that the same situation exists in the elderly. However, in the authors' experience, hypertension is a very rare cause of left ventricular failure in the elderly and by far the commonest causes of heart failure in this age group are tachyarrhythmias and myocardial infarction.

Assessment and investigations

In view of the above statements it will be clear that the assessment of the patient with raised levels of blood pressure is far from simple. Certainly no less than two blood pressure readings on separate occasions after at least five minutes rest are required before entertaining the diagnosis of hypertension. The age and sex of the patient are also vital. A thorough assessment of the general vascular status of the individual should be made, including palpation of the peripheral pulses and the optic fundi. The standing blood pressure should also be assessed, both at half a minute and three minutes.

Any significant fall in the standing blood pressure is a contra-indication to treatment. Similarly absence of target organ damage, such as normal retinal vessels, should make one very wary of instituting treatment.

The urine should be tested for the presence of sugar or albumen. An electrocardiogram (ECG) should be performed, and special note made of any arrhythmia, left ventricular hypertrophy and S–T change. A chest X-ray is necessary in order to assess the size of the left ventricle and any possible calcification of the cardiac valves. It will also help to exclude pulmonary lesions and the very rare case of aortic coarctation. The *serum electrolytes and blood urea and creatinine levels* will give some indication of the renal function and help to exclude hypovolaemic states and hyperaldosteronism.

Further investigations such as intravenous pyelograms, ultrasound scans and arteriography are only very rarely indicated. Reversible secondary causes of hypertension in the elderly are so rare that they can be virtually discounted.

Management

If the above criteria for the diagnosis of hypertension in the elderly are applied, there will be only a small number of patients that require active treatment and a rather larger group of people who should be monitored from time to time as to their blood pressure and cardiovascular status.

If the plan is to modify a patient's blood pressure, the objective should be to reduce the blood pressure slowly and by a modest amount so that recorded pressures are maintained in the range of 160/100 mmHg. Too great a reduction in pressure will lead to complications, such as postural hypotension, renal insufficiency or cerebral dysfunction that are unacceptable.

All chemical agents, and often even general advice about life style, have unwanted effects that will either harm the patient or make compliance impossible and, therefore, any regimen that is offered must be carefully planned.

General advice and patient self-help are very important in this condition. Many hypertensive patients are *overweight*. Sensible advice about diet may have a very beneficial effect both on the level of measured blood pressure and the patient's general well-being. Many problems in elderly people are either caused or exacerbated by obesity, but weight reduction in an elderly person is a very difficult goal to achieve. Years of inappropriate diet and inactivity are very hard to reverse. Despite this, however, it is encumbent on the general practitioner to make every effort to modify the situation. This will take both time and patience – factors which may be difficult to provide in a busy surgery. However, the practice nurse or health visitor can often help to reinforce the doctor's advice and provide continuing supervision. *Dietary advice* should be limited to calorie restriction and an increase in the dietary fibre. This will include limitation of both carbohydrate and fat. Worrying about niceties such as high and low density lipoproteins is quite unnecessary in the elderly. General increase in the elderly person's *physical activity* is important and will normally be limited to encouragement of more outside walking. This advice can be compromised by associated musculo-skeletal disorders, which will themselves require attention.

Drug treatment

If a decision has been made to modify a patient's blood pressure there is plenty of time to await the results of the general advice given above. *There is very rarely any urgency to treat hypertension.*

The first line of drug treatment is still with *simple diuretic agents.* The thiazide diuretics, such as hydrochlorothiazide (Hydrosaluric) 25–100 mg daily, or bendrofluazide (Neo-NaClex) 2.5–5 mg daily, are quite effective but must be given with potassium supplements e.g. Slow-K, Kloref. Alternatively a potassium sparing diuretic may be added, such as triamterene (Dytac) 50–100 mg daily, or amiloride (Midamor) 5–10 mg daily.

All diuretic agents may induce glucose intolerance and should not be used in diabetics. They may also lead to a rise in the serum uric acid level and induce clinical gout. There is no place for short-acting loop diuretics, such as bumetanide and frusemide, although these do have some hypotensive action.

The next line of drug treatment is with the *beta-adrenergic blocking agents*, of which there are a great many to choose from. There is probably no great advantage in using any particular drug, but propanolol, atenolol, oxprenolol and timolol are some of the most common agents in current use. The initial dosage should be small e.g. atenolol (Tenormin) 50 mg daily, propranolol (Inderal) 10 mg tds, timolol (Blocadren) 5 mg bd, as many elderly subjects are very sensitive to their effects. However, in some cases large doses of beta-blockers may be necessary to control the blood pressure. The chief unwanted effects of this group of drugs are bradycardia, glucose intolerance and bronchial muscle constriction. Thus their use in diabetics and particularly asthmatics may be hazardous.

In recent years *combination therapy with beta-blockers and diuretics* have become popular and they are indeed very effective. Very recent evidence suggests that the dosage of the diuretic in the combination tablet should be very small, since larger doses do not increase the anti-hypertensive effect but merely increase the risk of unwanted effects.

It has now been shown that the *calcium antagonist group of drugs*, of which nifedipine (Adalat) 5-10 mg tds is the best known, have a useful hypotensive action. These drugs do not appear to have an effect on either glucose metabolism or bronchial smooth muscle. Thus they may be safely used in diabetics and asthmatics. As with the beta-blockers they are useful in hypertensive patients who have angina as well. These agents do have an effect on cardiac conduction and should not be used in patients with any form of heart block.

The other main group of drugs that can be used in the elderly hypertensive are the *vasodilators*, such as prazosin and hydralazine. These drugs have a powerful hypotensive action and may cause a precipitous fall in the blood pressure, especially on standing. They should, therefore be used in very small doses initially e.g. hydralazine (Apresoline) 25 mg bd, prazosin (Hypovase) 0.5 mg bd initially and then 0.5 mg tds. Hydralazine, in particular, may cause a reflex tachycardia and, very rarely, an SLE-like syndrome, but this is not likely if the daily dose is kept below 100 mg.

In recent years increasing use has been made of the angiotensin-converting enzyme inhibitors (ACE), of which captopril (Capoten) is the best known example. These drugs inhibit the conversion of inactive Angiotensin I to the potent pressor agent Angiotensin II. They can be used to treat heart failure as well as hypertension. Captopril has been associated with severe side-effects due to its potent action in the elderly. These include rashes, proteinuria and marked hypotension, even when used in small doses. The more modern ACE inhibitor without the sulphydryl side chain, enalapril (Innovace), promises to be just as potent but should have less side-effects. At the present time there are very few elderly patients who will require ACE inhibitor treatment, but if they do the treatment should be initiated in hospital and then caried on in the community.

Drugs such as reserpine or bethanidine should not be used in the elderly. These drugs are associated with a large number of side-effects in this group of patients, including postural hypotension and depression. Although they have been useful in the past, the more modern agents are much safer.

It has already been pointed out that extensive investigations are not indicated in the elderly hypertensive. The main reason for this is that even if an underlying cause is found, for example renal artery stenosis or chronic renal disease, surgical correction will almost certainly not reverse the hypertension. Thus there is virtually no place for surgery in this condition.

Planned care

Once the diagnosis of hypertension has been established in an elderly person, continued follow-up should be planned, whether or not treatment is to be given. Initially a *monthly examination* should be undertaken, but as the problem settles down, three-monthly visits should be adequate. Clearly *associated problems*, such as diabetes, asthma or obesity, will need monitoring as well. If some groups of drugs are to be used, such as simple diuretics or beta-blockers, the *blood sugar and serum potassium levels* will need to be measured, monthly at first. A continued watch should be kept on the state of the vessels in the *optic fundi* and the routine *urinalysis*. From time to time an *ECG* should be recorded, especially if there are abnormalities when the patient is first seen. This will also be necessary if the patient develops angina or symptoms that could be attributable to heart block.

Many patients with raised blood pressure may be able to have their drug regimen modified as the blood pressure falls, and, indeed, *it may be possible to stop drug treatment altogether*. The question as to whether patients should be tailed off treatment when they reach the age of 75 years of age is still unanswered, but it would seem advisable to try and do this.

If a patient should develop a *stroke whilst on antihypertensive treatment, it is probably wise to reduce or stop this treatment,* since there is some evidence that patients following strokes do worse with treatment than without, whatever level their blood pressure. The majority of cerebrovascular accidents occurring during antihypertensive therapy are due to hypotension.

Most patients with elevated levels of blood pressure can be dealt with very satisfactorily in general practice, but on occasion it may be necessary to refer a patient to the local hospital specialist. *Indications for referral* would include a patient in whom the general practitioner finds difficulty in deciding whether they should be treated or not. A second opinion may also be required in patients who have some coexistent disease such as uncontrolled diabetes. Sometimes patients with coexistent angina may require more specialized tests, such as treadmill ECG monitoring, which are not generally available in general practice. There is no reason why the patient should not be returned to the care of the general practitioner once the investigations are completed or the drug regime stabilised.

SUMMARY

Measured levels of high blood pressure are frequently found in the elderly, but true hypertension which requires active treatment is not so common. Careful evaluation of the patient as a whole requires some expertise, since inappropriate treatment can be harmful and, on occasion, positively dangerous. Once measured high blood pressure has been detected long-term follow-up must be undertaken, whether or not active therapy is given. Investigation of high blood pressure in the elderly should be limited to simple blood analysis, chest X-ray and an ECG. More invasive tests are rarely required. Much can be done by initiating simple measures to affect lifestyle and dietary modification. Drug treatment of hypertension should be fairly straightforward and effective, providing that special care is taken in those patients with diabetes, asthma and conduction diseases of the heart.

ISCHAEMIC HEART DISEASE

Definition

Ischaemic heart disease is caused by narrowing of the coronary arteries by atheroma. Ischaemia leads to myocardial necrosis and replacement fibrosis as large lesions (>3.6 cm). Smaller lesions (<2 cm) are not due to ischaemia but are age-dependent and the result of focal myocarditis. Recently vasospasm as an alternative mechanism in the production of angina and myocardial infarction has been postulated in younger patients but there is no evidence that this occurs in the elderly.

Aetiology

Coronary atheroma starts early in life, but the clinical manifestations are rarely seen in youth and frequently occur in old age. It probably accounts for a third of all deaths in those over 65 years and exists in one quarter of the elderly in the community. About 4500 hospital beds in England and Wales are occupied daily by people over 65 with ischaemic heart disease.

The most important risk factor for ischaemic heart disease is numerical age itself. Because of the deposition of atheroma early in life it is likely that dietary habits, especially the high consumption of saturated fats, in childhood and adolescence constitute major risk factors. Cigarette smoking and untreated hypertension are known to increase the risk of ischaemic heart disease in middle life. Whether modification of dietary and smoking habits in later life beneficially affects the outcome of ischaemic heart disease is not known.

Clinical features

There are no special features in the clinical presentation of ischaemic heart disease in the elderly that do not occur in younger people. However, angina appears to be less of a problem in the elderly owing to the fact that their expectation of exercise is less than in the young. There have been several reports of painless myocardial infarction in the elderly, but in the authors' experience this is an unusual presentation.

Myocardial infarction in the elderly presents as in other age groups, but the incidence of post-infarction arrhythmias is higher, as is the mortality rate. The incidence of the post-myocardial syndrome of Dressler appears to be very low in the older age group.

Complications

Apart from the high incidence of arrhythmias following infarction, which affects the management (see below), the major problems following infarction concern the compromising of an old person's ability to continue to lead an independent life at home. This is especially true if the infarction has been extensive or if there is some *papillary muscle dysfunction* with left ventricular infarction. *Left ventricular aneurysm* formation and subsequent mural thrombus formation and systemic emboli do not appear to be a significant problem in the elderly. *Capsulitis of the shoulder* does not appear to become increasingly common after infarction with old age.

The major complications of angina in an elderly person concern his ability to continue to live an independent life alone, whether as a result of fear or reduced exercise tolerance.

Assessment and investigation

To some extent the intensity of investigation of an elderly person with angina will depend on his previous state of physical and mental health. Invasive investigations of someone with other disabling disease would be clearly meddlesome. However, all should have a full clinical examination of the heart and lungs and all should have a resting 12 lead ECG performed. The changes of the ECG should be assessed on the same criteria as used for younger people. The only age-related changes that occur on the ECG are a progressive shift of the electrical axis to the left, a prolongation of the

P–R interval and the appearance of T wave inversion in lead AVL in the absence of apparent heart disease.

Exercise testing using a treadmill may be indicated in more athletic old people and this will almost certainly require referral to a hospital specialist. The conventional treadmill exercise protocols are of little use and modified forms have to be used. This form of investigation should not be ruled out on the grounds of age alone, since coronary artery bypass surgery should certainly be considered for otherwise fit people up to the age of 75 if their angina is disabling and uncontrolled by drugs.

The diagnosis of myocardial infarction must be made on electrocardio-graphic as well as clinical and biochemical evidence. Any anginal pain that lasts more than 30 minutes and is not relieved by nitrates must be assumed to be due to infarction until proved otherwise. The electrocardiographic changes may not appear for 24 hours or so in some cases. The position and the thickness level of the infarction can be assessed by this method, but not its extent. The extent of the infarction can be judged on the length of the fever that occurs with muscle necrosis. The elevation of the peripheral white blood count (day 1) and the ESR (days 3–4) also help to assess the degree of muscle damage. The cardiac enzymes in the blood are also raised in proportion to the amount of muscle necrosis (SGOT: days 3–4; LDH: days 5–6).

Differential diagnosis

There are many other causes of chest pain that may mimic myocardial infarction. *Reflux oesophagitis* may be present as well and sometimes causes some confusion. In this condition the pain is often related to posture, and is usually described by the patient as burning and occurs in a vertical position behind the sternum. *Pulmonary embolism* may also produce retro-sternal pain, but there are usually signs of segmental collapse in the lung on auscultation and often a rub or a small pleural effusion.

Chest wall diseases, such as *Teitz's syndrome* of costochondritis, and *Bornholm disease* (Coxsackie B myalgia) are usually differentiated from infarction by the finding of localized chest wall or rib junction tenderness.

Pericarditis may be caused by infarction but is often due to a viral infection. The ECG changes are characteristic (see Figure 3.3) and a peri-cardial rub is usually heard. The cardiac enzymes are not elevated.

Dissection of the thoracic aorta usually starts off in the aortic root and may obliterate one or more of the coronary ostia, producing infarction. The pain is often referred to the back and the brachial pulses are unequal. The patient may succumb very quickly.

45

Management

In *myocardial infarction* the most important immediate decision that has to be made is whether to admit the patient to hospital or keep him at home. There is now abundant evidence that suggests that in an uncomplicated case home treatment is preferable. This presumes that the social circumstances in the home are satisfactory and that the family are prepared to accept responsibility. The principal complications that indicate admission to hospital are the appearance of arrhythmias, which can be controlled satisfactorily in a coronary care unit.

If it is decided to manage the patient at home the necessary blood tests and ECGs should be performed. The family will need counselling about the patient's condition and the likely outlook. Prolonged bed rest is no longer advisable after infarction, whatever its severity. A maximum of 24 hours should be spent in bed and thereafter gradual mobilization encouraged. The appearance of heart failure in the early stages does not appear to adversely affect the long term prognosis but will delay the process of remobilization. *Heart failure* should be treated aggressively, and the use of loop diuretics (frusemide (Lasix) 40–320 mg daily, bumetanide (Burinex) 1–5 mg daily) with either potassium supplementation or the addition of a potassium-sparing diuretic (amiloride (Midamor) 5–10 mg daily) is essential. Digoxin should never be given in this situation unless there is uncontrolled atrial fibrillation.

The occurrence of *arrhythmias* is an indication to consider transfer of the patient to hospital. Sometimes the patient will refuse admission and it is important to identify the disorder by means of electrocardiography. Ventricular arrhythmias of any type are best treated in the home by disopyramide 100 mg qds. This drug may cause a dry mouth and indigestion, and in old men retention of urine may be a problem. If these side-effects occur it is worth trying mexiletine 200 mg tds. Sometimes these arrhythmias are related to hypokalaemia and the electrolytes should be measured. A domiciliary visit by the consultant and general practitioner together can be extremely valuable in these circumstances.

Patient and family counselling

'Myocardial infarction' is a term that few lay people will understand. 'Heart attack' or 'coronary thrombosis' may be better understood, but are still likely to cause great fear and concern. The nature of the illness and the outlook for the patient, both in terms of survival and future activities, need to be explained extremely carefully, if necessary on more than one occasion.

Rehabilitation is important after infarction and every encouragement should be given to ensure return to normal and sometimes increased activities. Regular exercise may or may not be beneficial to survival, but a high level of fitness will certainly make that survival more rewarding. Excessive weight should be shed and most elderly patients will require a lot of help with dietary advice. Smoking of cigarettes should be banned. Sexual intercourse will be permissible after the first two weeks and patients need to be told this as few will ask the doctor. Alcohol in modest quantities can only help.

As far as survival and the possibility of re-infarction are concerned, it is probably best to take an optimistic line. One of the advantages of giving long-term prophylaxis (see below) is that patients will feel that something is being done to help them.

Long-term prevention of re-infarction

There have been several studies of both a variety of beta-blocking drugs and of agents that interfere with platelet aggregation in the long term prevention of re-infarction. The difficulty with these trials is that enormous numbers of patients are required for a long period of follow-up and this is prohibitively expensive. Results to date do suggest that the beta-blocking drugs propranolol, timolol, oxprenolol and alprenolol reduce the incidence of re-infarction and mortality in treated patients for up to two years. However, there are a significant number of patients who cannot be given these agents, e.g. diabetics and asthmatics, as well as those with atrioventricular block and bradycardia.

Trials of the anti-platelet drugs aspirin, aspirin and dipyridamole, and sulphinpyrazone have shown that the combination of aspirin 300 mg tds and dipyridamole (Persantin) 75 mg tds given in the first six months after infarction appeared to reduce the mortality. Sulphinpyrazone (Anturan) 400 mg bd also appeared to reduce re-infarction but did not affect the mortality rate. The evidence, therefore, for significant benefit accruing from the administration of these drugs is not all that strong. In view of the expense and aggravation of taking these drugs they cannot be recommended for the elderly on the evidence that we have to date.

ANGINA

The management of angina either occurring after myocardial infarction or *de novo* is similar to that in younger patients with some important differences. The first line of treatment is to give nitrates, either in the form of long-acting oral preparations, such as isosorbide dinitrate (Isordil) in a starting dose of 10 mg qds, increasing up to 40 mg qds, or to use the more expensive, but effective, transdermal nitrate patches (Transiderm-Nitro 5-10 mg daily). In addition these patients should be given escape trinitrin sublingually for the immediate treatment of an attack.

If these regimes fail to control the symptoms a beta-blocking agent should be added, such as propranolol (Inderal) 10 mg tds, atenolol (Tenormin) 50 mg daily or timolol (Blocadren) 5 mg bd. The doses of these drugs can be doubled or more if necessary. There are many patients to whom these drugs should not be given, including diabetics, asthmatics, and those with atrio-ventricular block, hypotension or cardiac failure.

For patients in whom beta-blockers are contra-indicated, a calcium antagonist, such as nifedipine (Adalat) 10-20 mg tds can be given. There is evidence that calcium antagonists and beta-blockers have a potentiating effect and in suitable patients they can be given together.

The great majority of the elderly will be well controlled by the above regime. In some patients failure to get adequate control of angina by these means should alert one to the possibility of bypass coronary surgery. This may be specially relevant if there is associated aortic valve disease as this can be replaced at the same time. Many doctors and patients may be alarmed by the thought of such major procedures, but, with the present state of the art and the excellent results that can be achieved, age itself should be no absolute contra-indication. Obviously careful assessment of the patient's general fitness and mental attitude is necessary. If the doctor feels that this route bears further consideration the patient should be referred to a cardiologist. The mortality rate for this operation is low and the results, as far as the relief of angina is concerned, are good. As in younger patients there is no good evidence that bypass grafting increases the long term survival rate.

CARDIAC DYSRHYTHMIAS

Definition

Cardiac dysrhythmias indicate any irregularity of the heart rhythm, whether these are occasional premature beats, sustained tachycardias or episodes of heart block and temporary cardiac standstill.

Aetiology

Cardiac muscle cells have the inherent ability to discharge electrical impulses, that is they can act as a pacemaker. This is known as 'rhythmicity'.

The ventricular muscle cells have the slowest rate of rhythmicity and those in the sino-atrial node the fastest. Thus in health the *sino-atrial node* assumes the role as the dominant *cardiac pacemaker*. This node is itself under the influence of sympathetic and parasympathetic nerve impulses, which respectively quicken and slow the rate of discharge of the node. From the sino-atrial node the electrical impulses travel through the atria to the *atrio-ventricular node* and thence to the main *bundle of His*. In the interventricular septum the His bundle divides into its main left and right branches which supply the respective ventricles. The left main bundle further subdivides into anterior and posterior fascicles.

Ageing is associated with degenerative changes in the *sino-atrial node* and the number of muscle cells can be shown to diminish with increasing age. This process may be accelerated in some diseases, such as rheumatic fever and ischaemic heart disease. When disease of the sino-atrial node occurs its role as the dominant pacemaker of the heart is embarrassed and other pacemakers may obtain dominance. This situation is known as the *sick sinus syndrome*.

There are other methods whereby the heart rhythm may be disturbed. Electrolyte disturbances, toxins and drugs may all make the heart muscle cells more irritable and allow spontaneous premature discharges. Heart muscle damage by infarction may cut off some of the normal electrical pathways as well as produce toxins that act as an irritant.

Ischaemic damage to the *atrio-ventricular node* may cause this area to malfunction and produce *heart block*. A similar situation may be produced by certain drugs, in particular digoxin.

Classification of cardiac dysrhythmias

Sick sinus syndrome
    Sinus bradycardia
    Loss of range of normal dynamic sinus rate
    Sinus arrest and sinus pauses
    Atrial fibrillation and flutter

'Irritant' dysrhythmias
    Supraventricular premature complexes
    Supraventricular tachycardias (atrial and junctional)
    Ventricular premature complexes
    Ventricular tachycardia, fibrillation and flutter

Re-entry tachycardias
    Atrial fibrillation
    Supraventricular tachycardias

Heart block
1°,2°,3° atrioventricular block

Symptomatology of cardiac dysrhythmias

A large number of symptoms referable both to the heart and central nervous system may be produced by dysrhythmias. Although it is often difficult to establish a direct correlation between a dysrhythmia and symptoms such as dizziness, vertigo, fits, faints and falls, chest pain and palpitations in the elderly, these symptoms may often be due to a disordered action of the heart rhythm. In addition dysrhythmias are an important cause of breathlessness and chest pain.

In general terms rapid dysrhythmias cause chest pain and shortness of breath and slow rhythms cause dizziness, fits, faints and falls. Palpitations may be caused by either slow or fast heart rates, but it is important to determine exactly what the patient means by palpitation (see Section 2).

The difficulty in interpreting symptoms, such as dizziness and syncope in the elderly, is that there are many causes of these, of which dysrhythmias are only one. From a practical point of view, if the symptoms are serious and a dysrhythmia can be demonstrated, then it is wise to treat it even if a direct correlation cannot be shown.

Investigation and assessment

Clinical examination will demonstrate a disorderly heart rhythm but will rarely point to the exact diagnosis. Similarly a resting 12 lead ECG will demonstrate established dysrhythmias, such as *atrial fibrillation* and *heart block*, but it will usually fail to elucidate the paroxysmal rhythm disturbances, which often cause more in the way of clinical symptoms.

The introduction of *ambulatory dynamic electrocardiography* by Holter in the early 1960s has made possible the elucidation of paroxysmal dysrhythmias, and in more recent times has allowed us to quantify the rhythm disturbance with great accuracy. Ambulatory ECGs should now be available in every district hospital. The conventional method of using a reel-to-reel tape is still the best method of doing ambulatory monitoring, but there are other simpler devices that can be played back through a standard ECG machine. Although it is tempting to use these devices in general practice, they lack a lot of the flexibility and accuracy of the much more expensive 'Holter' systems and are not to be generally recommended.

Ambulatory ECG recordings will demonstrate over 90% of all dysrhythmias on a single 24 hour tape, and, therefore, further tapes will only produce an extra 5% yield since it is only possible to elucidate 98% of arrhythmias after five days of continuous recordings. It is essential for the patient to fill in a diary of events throughout the period of recording and these can be more carefully analysed by the technician to try and correlate events with ECG abnormalities. It is important for the elderly patient to undergo a full programme of activities during the period of recording in order to see what happens to the heart rhythm during a normal period of activity.

The spectrum of dysrhythmias that are found on ambulatory monitoring of healthy old people is quite wide. Therefore care needs to be put on the interpretation of the findings in symptomatic elderly people. With this in mind every effort should be made to make sure that the events diary is completed as fully and accurately as possible. The incidence of rhythm abnormalities that one might expect to find in healthy people at the age of 70 years is shown in Table 3.1. It must be remembered that although these subjects have been judged to be healthy, many of the rhythm disturbances that they showed were associated with symptoms, such as palpitations and dizziness.

Table 3.1 Approximate percentage of rhythm disturbances found in apparently healthy old people

Rhythm disturbance	Percentage
Sinus arrhythmia	15
Sinus bradycardia (<60 bpm)	10
Sinus bradycardia (<40 bpm)	2
Sinus arrest and sinus pauses	0–1
Atrial fibrillation	8–12
Atrial and junctional premature complexes	40–45
Supraventricular tachys	1–3
Ventricular premature complexes (<10/hr)	55–60
Ventricular premature complexes (>100/hr)	10–15
Paroxysmal ventricular tachy	2–4

Thus interpretation of an ambulatory tape has to take into account the expected 'normal' pattern of dysrhythmias in any particular age group and the symptoms that are recorded in the events diary. Old people tend to tolerate extremes of heart rate rather badly. Heart rates above 140 per minute and below 40 per minute will almost certainly produce symptoms and should be regarded as abnormal. Similarly the finding of *ventricular premature complexes at rates of greater than 100 per hour is probably abnormal*, especially if they are associated with multifocal and paired complexes or occur in salvoes of three or four beats together. On the other hand *isolated ventricular premature complexes* or *supraventricular premature complexes* can probably be regarded as within normal limits.

Ambulatory tape recordings can also be useful if they show a normal rhythm in the presence of 'cardiac' symptoms described in the diary as these patients can be reassured that their symptoms have no cardiac basis. Relatively minor abnormalities on the tape can also suggest the occurrence of a more sinister dysrhythmia, for example, very frequent *atrial premature beats* may be associated with *paroxysmal atrial fibrillation*, and complex and frequent *ventricular ectopic beats* may be associated with *paroxysmal ventricular tachycardia* or *flutter*. The detection of intermittent degrees of atrioventricular block on an otherwise normal tape may suggest that a patient with infrequent syncopal attacks may be having periods of *complete heart block*.

Management of dysrhythmias

Atrial fibrillation is a dysrhythmia frequently found in the elderly and quite often is paroxysmal in nature. This makes its detection difficult without ambulatory taping. *Paroxysmal atrial fibrillation* inevitably progresses to *established atrial fibrillation* in time unless it is treated. It is clearly better to try and keep the patient in permanent sinus rhythm in order to maximize the cardiac output by preserving the atrial kick, and to abolish the symptoms of palpitations and breathlessness that these patients get when they go into paroxysmal atrial fibrillation with an associated rapid ventricular rate.

The best drug to control *paroxysmal atrial fibrillation* is amiodarone. This drug has been associated with a large number of side-effects, but these are minimized if the dose is kept low over long periods. The starting dose of amiodarone (Cordarone X) is 600 mg daily in three divided doses for two weeks, then reducing to 400 mg daily for a further fortnight and then to a maintenance dose of 200 mg daily. The side-effect profile of this drug is rather alarming and includes shaking of a rather parkinsonian nature, disturbances of thyroid and liver function and, rarely, pulmonary infiltration. All these side-effects are dose related and should not occur to any significant degree if the dose is kept low, as described above. Ideally the serum level of the drug should be monitored every three to six months and this can be done by sending a small serum sample to the Guy's Poisons Centre at New Cross Hospital, London. All patients on amiodarone develop deposition of the drug in the cornea, since it is insoluble in normal saline, but this has not been associated with any visual symptoms over the 15 years that the drug has been in use. Patients on this drug also may develop photosensitive rashes on exposed parts, but this is not common and is an idiosyncratic reaction and not dose-related. The results of amiodarone treatment for paroxysmal atrial fibrillation are extremely good, and at least 85% of patients should be controlled in sinus rhythm over long periods.

The reason for this detailed explanation of amiodarone treatment is that it is the best drug that we have at the present time that is available in general practice. Other anti-arrhythmic drugs, such as quinidine, verapamil and disopyramide are much less effective and are also associated with significant side-effects. Newer drugs such as flecainide are not yet available in general practice and do not appear to be so effective as amiodarone anyway.

Established atrial fibrillation is often associated with a rapid ventricular rate and will thus give rise to symptoms in the elderly. The treatment of choice in these patients is still with digoxin, unless the atrial fibrillation is due to re-entry through accessory pathways as in the *Wolff-Parkinson-White syndrome* which is extremely rare in the elderly. The dose of digoxin needs to be kept low (0.0625–0.125 mg/day), especially if there is any impairment of renal function. If the ventricular rate is still not controlled during exercise on this regimen, the concurrent administration of a beta-blocking agent will usually be effective providing there is no history of asthma or diabetes. An agent such as pindolol (Visken), which has a degree of partial agonist activity, is a good choice to blunt cardio-acceleration due to exercise whilst not reducing the resting heart rate. Amiodarone may also be used to control the ventricular rate in established atrial fibrillation. Some untreated patients with *atrial fibrillation* will have an associated high degree of *atrio-ventricular block* and consequent bradycardia. If this gives rise to symptoms of syncope, they should be paced.

Atrial premature complexes, unless associated with paroxysmal atrial fibrillation or flutter, require no treatment.

Ventricular premature complexes occurring at rates of less than 100 per hour are probably benign and, unless they cause symptoms of palpitations, do not require treatment. Perhaps surprisingly tea and coffee consumption in the elderly appear to have no effect on these dysrhythmias.

Frequent and *complex ventricular premature complexes* are more likely to give rise to symptoms and may be associated with an increased risk of *ventricular tachycardia, flutter and fibrillation*. There is thus a significant risk of sudden death. At the present time the hard evidence for this statement is lacking and, therefore, in an asymptomatic patient no treatment need be given. If treatment is to be given there are a large number of drugs that can be used, all of which may have unacceptable side-effects in the elderly. Quinidine, mexiletine (Mexitil) and tocainide (Tonocard) are moderately effective and are generally well-tolerated in the elderly. Disopyramide (Norpace, Rythmodan) are quite effective at controlling ventricular dysrhythmias, but give rise to unacceptable side-effects, particularly in elderly men (urinary retention, dry mouth, indigestion, constipation and glaucoma). Flecainide (Tambocor) is quite effective but is not available at the present time in general practice. Amiodarone is probably the best drug available to the general practitioner currently.

Bundle branch block is not strictly a dysrhythmia, but is quite commonly found as an incidental finding in the elderly (5–10%). In the elderly it is due to fibrosis of the conducting system rather than due to ischaemia. The importance of its recognition lies in the finding of *bi-fascicular block*, when two of the three branches of the conducting system are blocked, for example, the right bundle branch and the anterior fascicle of the left bundle. This can be recognized easily from the resting ECG. *Bi-fascicular block* ultimately progresses to *complete heart block*, usually with an associated very slow ventricular rhythm which gives rise to syncope. These patients should be considered for permanent *cardiac pacing*.

Atrioventricular block. The prevalence of a PR interval greater than 0.22 seconds increases with age and will be found in 5–10% of the elderly. This *first degree heart block* is not associated with clinical heart disease and when found as an isolated abnormality does not adversely affect the prognosis and requires no treatment. *Higher degrees of atrioventricular block* are rarely found in apparently healthy old people. Complete heart block is nearly always symptomatic, producing syncopal attacks and extreme lethargy. *All patients with complete heart block require permanent pacing* irrespective of their symptomatic status since the prognosis, even in the very old, is improved.

Pacemakers

Any bradycardic situation from whatever cause requires treatment with a permanent on-demand pacemaker. The rate of *pacemaker implantation* in Great Britain has, in the past, been much lower than in virtually all other developed countries. This fact is in part due to the previously poor availability of ambulatory heart monitoring and to some extent due to the conservatism of doctors to treat the *sick sinus syndrome* with pacing in the belief that it was a benign condition. From a mortality point of view sinus node disease is unlikely to lead to sudden death, but sinus pauses of greater than 2 seconds are likely to lead to significant symptoms of severe dizziness and syncope. Similarly *sinus bradycardia* may lead to considerable impairment of an elderly person's exercise tolerance. Thus the tendency recently is for more pacemakers to be inserted in the elderly with these conditions.

The correct pacemaker implantation rate is likely to be at least 1–2 per thousand population per year. Thus every general practice will have some patients with a permanent pacemaker in the future. It is, therefore, important that general practitioners should be able to recognize pacing complexes on the ECG and to understand the simple principles of capturing and correct sensing. The recent advent of dual chamber pacing systems has made the situation more complex.

A permanent pacing spike can be clearly seen on the ECG as the only waveform that is completely vertical and this is followed by a wide QRST complex. The absence of this wide QRST complex indicates failure to capture, and this situation requires immediate referral to the local pacemaker service as the patient is in great danger of reverting to his pre-pacing bradycardic state. Correct sensing is more difficult to interpret, but with on-demand pacing systems that are currently used the interposition of a normal cardiac beat will suppress the pacing beat and the vertical pacing spike will be delayed on the ECG. In addition to loss of capture and failure to sense accurately, other pacemaker arrhythmias may occur. These are most commonly pacemaker suppression by external electromagnetic radiation, although most modern units revert to the fixed rate mode of pacing in this situation. Unipolar pacemakers may be suppressed by excessive myopotentials, but this problem does not occur if bipolar electrodes are used. The pacing rhythm may also be suppressed by paroxysmal tachycardias and an anti-arrhythmic drug will have to be given. If there is any doubt about a pacemaker function the patient should be referred to the local pacing clinic, where routine checking should be carried out anyway. It is impossible to measure the pacemaker discharge rate by means of examining an ECG and this assessment must be made by sophisticated electronic analysis.

HEART FAILURE

Heart failure is a syndrome caused by an abnormality of the heart, which can produce a characteristic pattern of haemodynamic, renal, neural and hormonal responses. Heart failure may be *acute* or *chronic* and may produce a state of *circulatory collapse.*

The body's response to heart failure

The affected ventricle hypertrophies.

Fluid is redistributed within the circulation and is accompanied by vasoconstriction and sodium retention by the kidney which increases the circulatory volume. There is an increased filling pressure in the affected ventricle which maintains the cardiac output to some degree on the basis of the Starling's Law.

The sympathetic nervous and the renin-angiotensin systems are activated and increased plasma levels of aldosterone and vasopressin occur.

There is a change in local blood flow in certain areas. Renal blood flow is reduced and there is an increase in the peripheral vascular resistance.

Symptoms

Tiredness is an early symptom of *chronic heart failure* and this may be generalized or localized to the legs, as a result of reduced muscle blood flow. Oedema of the legs is also a common symptom of this condition. In bedridden patients the oedema will occur in the sacral area. The sudden onset of marked breathlessness is a feature of *acute heart failure*. This is caused by pulmonary oedema. Cyanosis and peripheral vasoconstriction may also occur in *acute heart failure*.

Circulatory collapse or 'cardiogenic shock' is a serious condition and is usually caused by myocardial infarction. There is a profound fall in blood pressure, peripheral vasoconstriction and a fall in urine output.

Principal causes of heart failure in the elderly

Myocardial ischaemia and infarction

Cardiac dysrhythmias, especially paroxysmal atrial fibrillation with rapid ventricular rates

Cardiomyopathies: amyloidosis
                      alcoholic
                      thyroid disease

Valvular disease: principally aortic and mitral

Drugs: beta-blockers
         anti-arrhythmic drugs
         calcium channel antagonists

The diagnosis and investigation of heart failure

The diagnosis of heart failure alone is inadequate. It is vital to determine the cause accurately. However, in the acute situation the general practitioner must institute treatment immediately and the investigation of the cause will be a secondary procedure. Apart from a careful clinical examination of the heart by means of the stethoscope it will be necessary to obtain a resting electrocardiogram and a chest X-ray. These simple investigations will point to the vast majority of the principal causes of heart failure listed above. Simple blood investigations, such as a full blood count, urea and electrolyte estimation are essential. Thyroid disease may be difficult to diagnose clinically in an elderly patient and it will be necessary to perform the thyroid function tests.

Quite a lot of information can be determined from clinical examination of the heart, but if significant valvular disease is suspected it will be necessary to refer the patient to the local district general hospital for further evaluation by means of an echocardiogram. This is important as surgical correction of aortic and mitral valve stenosis and incompetence is increasingly being performed in the elderly. Numerical age on its own is no longer a contra-indication to major heart surgery if the patient is otherwise physically and mentally healthy, and the results of valve replacement surgery in carefully chosen patients up to the age of 80 are very satisfactory.

Since transient and established cardiac dysrhythmias are a major cause of heart failure in the elderly it is essential to demonstrate these, especially if there are no other obvious causes for the failure. Paroxysmal atrial fibrillation is particularly difficult to demonstrate since the dysrhythmia may have ceased by the time that the patient is seen by the general practitioner. It is important to have a high index of suspicion in these cases; there may be a history obtainable that points to 'palpitations', or the pulse and ECG may show premature atrial contractions. In these cases it will be necessary to refer the patient for 24 hour ambulatory electrocardiography (DCG). Over 90% of significant dysrhythmias can be excluded by a single 24 hour tape recording. The importance of correctly diagnosing cardiac dysrhythmias as a cause of heart failure cannot be overstressed since the long-term management is different.

Myocardial ischaemia and infarction are important causes of heart failure and can, to a large extent, be evaluated by serial ECGs. However, it may be necessary to refer some patients for further investigation by exercise ECG if there is any doubt about the diagnosis or if there is to be some consideration of surgical coronary artery bypass grafting. Despite the pressures being generated by the increasing need for this operation in younger people, most cardiac surgeons are happy to consider this operation in older people up to the age of 75 years, if the symptoms are uncontrollable by drugs.

In many old people cardiac failure can be precipitated by an acute chest infection or by the exacerbation of chronic lung disease, although this will not occur in the absence of significant heart disease. However, it is a truism to say that any acute attack of breathlessness in an elderly patient who has no history of lung disease is almost certainly due to cardiac failure.

Less common causes of heart failure are subacute bacterial endocarditis and rupture of an aortic or mitral valve cusp. Valvular rupture is often caused by bacterial endocarditis, but may occur after myocardial infarction or spontaneously. Both these conditions are to be suspected if there are changing murmurs associated with quite severe degrees of heart failure.

MANAGEMENT OF HEART FAILURE

Acute heart failure

The conventional treatment, whereby the patient is sat up in bed and given morphine 5–10 mg or diamorphine 5 mg intravenously, is still the best emergency treatment. The additional use of intravenous frusemide (Lasix) 40–80 mg or bumetanide (Burinex) 1–2 mg is advisable. Both the opiates and the diuretics act immediately by their vasodilator action. In addition the opiates reduce the anxiety that accompanies acute heart failure. The powerful diuretic action of frusemide (Lasix) and bumetanide (Burinex) is a secondary, but important, action.

In some cases it may be difficult to differentiate acute bronchial from acute cardiac asthma, and in these it is better not to give an opiate since these have a respiratory depressant action. In this situation intravenous aminophylline 250–500 mg should be given. In both cases oxygen administration will be helpful, if it is available.

More recently it has been shown that short-acting nitrates, such as glyceryl trinitrate (GNT) sublingually or GTN oral spray (Nitrolingual) have a useful vasodilator effect in acute heart failure. In the future these agents may replace more traditional treatment.

If there is a cardiac dysrhythmia that has precipitated the heart failure it is important to treat this as well. If established atrial fibrillation is present and the ventricular rate is high digoxin should be given in a loading dose of 0.5 mg orally. Intravenous digoxin should not be given at home unless under ECG control, and then with great caution.

Acute heart failure can be very satisfactorily treated at home and does not constitute a reason for admission to hospital unless there is a difficult dysrhythmia to treat, or the patient does not respond to the management outlined above.

Circulatory collapse

The management of circulatory collapse depends to some extent on the clinical diagnosis of the case. The majority of cases are due to acute myocardial infarction. In this situation the pain should be controlled with intravenous morphine or diamorphine. The use of inotropic drugs will have an adverse effect in the presence of acute myocardial infarction and generally these drugs should not be used, except as a last resort. There is little more that can be achieved by treating the patient at home and this situation is an indication for immediate hospital admission.

Chronic heart failure

It is important to identify the cause of the failure. Hypertension is very rarely a cause of heart failure in the elderly. The failure is much more likely to be due to ischaemic heart disease or some dysrhythmia. Valve disease and some cardiomyopathies or drug-induced heart failures are also important causes of heart failure in the elderly and should be clearly identified and treated as far as possible.

The management of chronic heart failure will depend on its severity and can be usefully subdivided in the following way:

Mild

Stop added salt and alcohol intake. Encourage weight reduction if this is a problem. Stop smoking and treat the patient with a mild diuretic, such as a thiazide with either potassium supplementation or in combination with a potassium-sparing diuretic. There are numerous suitable drugs currently available, but the author's preferences are for either bendrofluazide with potassium added to the tablet (Neo-NaClex-K) or for hydrochlorothiazide with the combination of amiloride (Moduretic).

Moderate

In this situation it will be necessary to give a stronger diuretic if the above measures have been inadequate to control the failure. Replacement of the thiazide drug should be with a loop diuretic, such as frusemide (Lasix) or bumetanide (Burinex) and the dosage should be adjusted to achieve the desired clinical effect. These drugs are powerful excretors of potassium and should be given with adequate potassium supplementation or with a potassium-sparing drug such as triamterene (Dytac), spironolactone (Aldactone) or amiloride (Midamor). Several combination preparations are now available to simplify drug-taking. The problems with all these powerful drugs in the elderly are that they may cause incontinence and are likely to produce some glucose intolerance.

Severe

In this situation it is necessary to increase the dose of the loop diuretics. The doses used may be quite large, for example old people can tolerate at least 500 mg frusemide (Lasix) a day, although the blood urea level may rise quite sharply on this dose.

Digoxin is the only widely used inotropic drug available at the present time, and even in the absence of atrial fibrillation it may benefit some patients. In the elderly considerable care has to be taken to make sure that the digoxin dose is controlled to avoid toxicity, especially if there is impairment of renal function.

The introduction of a wide variety of vasodilators has further increased our ability to manage severe heart failure. The nitrates, GTN and isosorbide dinitrate (Isordil), have some short-term effect on helping severe heart failure but their effect is not maintained in the long-term. Similarly hydralazine (Aspresoline) has the same shortcomings. The angiotensin converting enzymes (ACE) are now the most widely prescribed vasodilators in severe heart failure. Captopril (Capoten) is probably too toxic for widespread use in the elderly and enalapril (Innovace) is currently the drug of choice. All the ACE inhibitors have a worsening effect on renal failure and may increase the plasma potassium concentration. This makes them unsuitable for use in many old people and at the same time potassium supplements must be stopped. The ACE inhibitors may also precipitate a dramatic fall in cardiac output in some patients and it is essential for this treatment to be started in hospital: once tolerance has been established their use is safe in the community.

SUMMARY

Cardiac failure is an eminently suitable problem that can be treated in general practice. It is essential to diagnose the cause of the failure accurately, and as far as possible to correct it. This may involve investigations and treatment that are only available in hospital. However, the acute management of heart failure and its long-term control are generally well able to be managed by the general practitioner at home.

BONE DISEASE OF AGEING

Bone is composed of living cells and a matrix of collagen upon which bone salts are deposited. There is a constant replacement of both cancellous and cortical bone throughout life. Even in the old there are very large exchanges of calcium between the intestine, the kidneys and bones. Changes in the reformation and resorption of bone underly the diseases that occur in the adult skeleton. The maximum amount of bone in the body occurs in the fourth decade. After the age of 45 years there is a gradual loss of bone from the skeleton, the rate of loss being faster in women than in men. The composition of bone is affected by many factors including oestrogen levels, the action of parathyroid hormone, calcium and vitamin D intake, cortico-steroid levels and, very importantly, immobilization.

Bone disease may present in three different ways:
Pain
Fracture
Immobility

These presenting symptoms will be described in more detail under the headings of each major disease of bone found in the elderly. For practical purposes there are four main diseases of bone that may occur in combination and are found frequently in the population at home:
Osteoporosis
Osteomalacia
Paget's disease
Malignant disease

Osteoporosis

Osteoporosis is a reduction in bone mass, which is of normal composition.

Aetiology

This is the most common disorder of bone in the elderly and affects at least 20% of women by the age of about 70 years. After the age of about 45 years there is a progressive loss of bone from the skeleton in both men and women (Figure 3.5).

Thus people with a *small bone mass in middle age*, especially women, may lose sufficient bone with advancing years to cause osteoporosis in old age. There may be other factors that cause acceleration of this bone loss. This is seen in post-menopausal women where the reduced oestrogen levels result

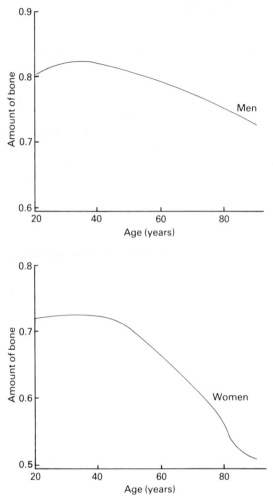

Figure 3.5 Schematic representation of bone loss with age (from Martin (1981), *Problems in Geriatric Medicine*, p. 154 (Lancaster: MTP Press))

in increased sensitivity to parathormone and/or vitamin D. This in turn leads to increased bone resorption and a greater calcium requirement.

Increased bone loss also occurs with *corticosteroid excess*. This is most often seen in the elderly who are given steroid drugs for the control of conditions such as rheumatoid arthritis, asthma, skin disease and polymyalgia rheumatica. Steroids reduce the intestinal absorption of calcium and probably reduce the tubular resorption of calcium in the kidney.

Post-menopausal women are particularly sensitive to steroid treatment since there is further depression of oestrogen output due to the steroid suppression of the pituitary/adrenal axis.

Immobilization also causes osteoporosis. This is probably due to venous stasis and consequent bone resorption. The resulting osteoporosis may be localized, as in splintage of a fracture, during immobility after a stroke or with joint disease. Generalized osteoporosis will occur in patients who are chair or bed bound and is seen to occur quite rapidly in younger people who are exposed to weightlessness, for example in space travel.

A low calcium intake and absorption will also cause osteoporosis. Foods low in calcium form the staple diet of many old people. Patients who have had a gastrectomy or who have intestinal ischaemia will fail to absorb adequate calcium. Dietary insufficiency of calcium also occurs in alcoholics.

Clinical features

Many patients will have no symptoms at all. Fractures are common and may be the presenting feature of the disease. These occur most frequently in the proximal femur and vertebral bodies. Backache is one of the commonest symptoms and may be chronic and severe. The pain is worsened by movement of the spine, especially rotational movement, and is relieved by rest. Spinal deformity may occur due to vertebral wedging and compression. In advanced cases there may be considerable loss of height. Thoracic kyphosis may be severe enough to cause respiratory embarrassment. In advanced cases the kyphosis may be severe enough to cause pain due to impingement of the lower ribs on the pelvis (the 'kissing rib syndrome').

Investigation and differential diagnosis

Osteoporosis may be difficult to distinguish from osteomalacia and, indeed, the two conditions may occur together. The early stages of osteoporosis are difficult to recognize, and the radiological changes are the most useful indicator. Lateral thoracic and lumbar spine X-rays show a lack of contrast between the vertebrae and the surrounding tissues and intervertebral discs. The upper and lower margins of the vertebral body will be seen to be more radio-opaque than the centre and it may be possible to see accentuated vertical trabeculation at the expense of the horizontal trabeculae. The vertebrae may be deformed and in advanced cases there is anterior wedging and later compression of the vertebral bodies.

Biochemical tests are not helpful in the diagnosis of osteoporosis, as the plasma calcium, phosphate and alkaline phosphatase are normal. These tests help to differentiate osteoporosis from osteomalacia, since in the latter condition there is usually a rise in the alkaline phosphatase and phosphate and a lowering of the serum calcium (Table 3.2).

Table 3.2 Biochemical findings in bone disease (from Martin, *Problems in Geriatric Medicine*, p. 161 (Lancaster: MTP Press))

Disease	Calcium	Phosphate	Alkaline phosphatase	Acid phosphatase
Osteomalacia	N or ↓	N or ↑	N or ↑	N
Osteoporosis	N	N	N	N
Carcinoma of the prostate	N	N	↑	↑
Myeloma	N	N	N	N
Paget's	N	N	↑	N
Other 2° carcinoma	N	N	↑	N

The urinary calcium and hydroxyproline levels may be raised in osteoporosis, but these tests are not specific.

Bone biopsy may help in the investigation of a difficult case. This investigation, using sections of undecalcified bone, requires considerable expertise and is not generally available.

Management

The objective of management of the elderly patient with osteoporosis is to lessen pain and deformity and to prevent fractures.

The most important preventative factor in osteoporosis is to *maintain mobility*. Continued stress on bones will diminish the rate of bone resorption and continued exercise will have the other beneficial effect of keeping the elderly fitter both mentally and physically. This may be difficult when there is pain from joint or muscle disease and analgesic or anti-inflammatory drugs may be of help in some people. Similarly treatment of cardiac or respiratory disease may be necessary. After strokes or other neurological disorders physiotherapy may be necessary.

It is important to recognize the potentially fast bone losers, whether these be post-menopausal women, those on steroids, or those who start elderly life with a small bone mass. Adequate dietary calcium should be ensured and, if necessary, calcium supplements can be given in a dose of 800–1200 mg daily. If there is evidence of calcium malabsorption, as in those on steroid treatment, the administration of vitamin D 50 000 units twice weekly will help.

The management of post-menopausal women is difficult. Those with small bone mass should probably be given small doses of oral vitamin D and cyclical oestrogens, such as ethinyl oestradiol 0.025 mg daily for three weeks out of four. This will cause withdrawal bleeding which requires careful explanation to the patient. Most women will be prepared to accept this. Patients with heart disease or a history of thrombo-embolism should not receive oestrogens.

Anabolic steroids have been used for the prevention and treatment of oestoporosis but there is little evidence that they are of help.

Patients receiving calcium or vitamin D supplementation should be periodically screened for biochemical disturbances, especially hypercalcaemia.

The management of pain, especially backache, may be difficult. Most respond to adequate analgesia, local heat or infra-red radiation, but in some rest may be necessary. Bed rest should be limited to minimum possible time in view of the risk of immobility noted above.

Osteomalacia

Osteomalacia is a generalized disease of bone and is characterized by decalcification of the skeleton in which the bony matrix is normal.

Aetiology

Osteomalacia occurs in at least 5% of people over the age of 70 years in Great Britain. It is caused by lack of vitamin D and is, therefore, an important and correctable disorder.

The two major sources of vitamin D are dietary intake and the action of ultraviolet light upon the skin (Figure 3.6).

The dietary vitamin occurs as vitamin D2 where it is found in fish oils, eggs, milk and cereals. In Great Britain margarine is fortified with vitamin D and in the USA milk is also fortified. Hence malabsorption states and obstructive jaundice will lead to dietary vitamin D lack.

Vitamin D3 is formed in the skin by the action of ultraviolet light. Interference with sunlight through atmospheric pollution will drastically cut down the amount of ultraviolet radiation. In the elderly the most common lack of exposure to ultraviolet is due to their long established habit of not going out into the sunlight and, if they do, wearing a lot of clothes and broad-brimmed hats.

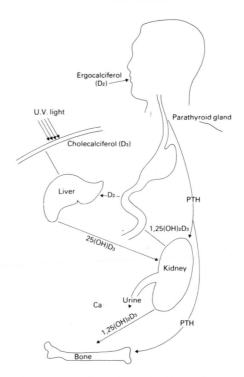

Figure 3.6 Schematic representation of vitamin D metabolism (from Martin (1981) *Problems in Geriatric Medicine*, p. 157 (Lancaster: MTP Press))

Vitamin D metabolism may be upset in other ways:

Chronic liver disease will produce impairment of the hydroxylation of vitamin D3 to 25-hydroxycholecalciferol.

Chronic renal disease may impair the I-hydroxylation of 25-hydroxycholecalciferol to 1.25 dihydroxycholecalciferol (1.25-OH-D3). 1.25–OH2-D3 is believed to be the active metabolite and regulates calcium absorption from the gut and the resorption of calcium from the renal tubules.

Anticonvulsant drugs also interfere with vitamin D metabolism and cause osteomalacia.

Clinical features

Bone pain is the commonest feature of osteomalacia. It may be generalized and persistent. It is probably caused by tendon strain on soft tender bone. Pain can be elicited by pressure on affected bones.

Muscular weakness is an important sign of osteomalacia and may take the form of a proximal myopathy, affecting both shoulder and hip girdles. This weakness gives rise to a characteristic 'waddling' gait and there is often difficulty in climbing stairs and combing the hair.

Fractures may be the presenting feature of osteomalacia and these may occur most frequently in the proximal femur, the ribs and scapulae.

Bony deformity may occur and usually takes the form of kyphosis due to compression of the vertebral bodies.

Investigation and differential diagnosis

The major disorder to differentiate from osteomalacia is osteoporosis. The bone pain and tenderness of osteomalacia may also be mistaken for secondary malignant disease affecting bones.

The radiological changes of osteomalacia show characteristic pseudofractures (Looser's zones) usually occurring in the ribs, scapulae, pelvis, femoral neck and the tibia. Looser's zones consist of bands of decalcification occurring obliquely or at right angles to the bone surfaces. These appear as incomplete fractures. Other changes may mimic osteoporosis, such as crush fractures and biconcavity of the vertebral bodies.

The biochemical changes of osteomalacia are variable but characteristic. The plasma calcium level may be normal or decreased; the serum alkaline phosphatase and phosphate levels are usually raised (Table 3.2) and the urinary excretion of calcium is low.

It is now possible to measure the serum 25-hydroxycholecalciferol level in some centres and this is reduced in osteomalacia. Iliac crest bone biopsy is also diagnostic of osteomalacia, but requires expert histological examination of an undecalcified sample of bone.

Management

The objective of management is to identify those old people at risk and to treat those with the disease before major symptoms of pain, immobility and fracture become a problem.

The recognition of potential sufferers from the disease means that a history of dietary intake and sunlight exposure should be taken of all old people seen in the home or general practical surgery. It is even more important to bear the diagnosis in mind when people complain of bone pain and diminishing ability to climb stairs or generally poor mobility.

Patients on long-term anticonvulsant therapy should be routinely screened annually for biochemical abnormality.

Once the disease is recognized treatment is with calciferol BP 1.25 mg daily and a calcium supplement (800–1200 mg daily). There is some evidence that alphacalcidol (One-Alpha) 1 mg daily may be preferable as it has a faster action and shorter half-life than calciferol and thus it is more easy to avoid, and reverse, the hypercalcaemia that may occur with vitamin D treatment. In the first week or so of treatment the bony pain of osteomalacia may actually get worse, but after that there is progressive reduction in pain and increase in muscle strength. It is important to monitor the serum calcium and alkaline phosphatase levels weekly for the first month or two of treatment since hypercalcaemia may occur and this is potentially dangerous. The most common symptoms of hypercalcaemia are nausea and confusion. When the biochemical levels return to near normal the dose of vitamin D can be reduced to maintenance levels (125 mg once or twice daily).

Paget's disease (osteitis deformans)

In Paget's disease there is uncontrolled osteoclastic resorption of bone and this is followed by chaotic deposition of new bone. This leads to bone thickening and considerable deformity of the skeleton with increased vascularity.

Aetiology

Paget's disease of bone is very rare before the age of 40 years and increases in frequency after the age of 60 years, after which time about 3% of the population are affected. By the ninth decade the incidence is of the order of 11%.

Paget's disease appears to be rather more common in men than in women. The disease is more prevalent in races from Western Europe and less common in Scandinavia, Africa and China. It is particularly prevalent in the mill towns of Lancashire where it affects some 6–8% of men and women over the age of 55 years.

It is now thought that the disease is due to infection with a slow virus.

Clinical features

Paget's disease can involve any bone or combination of bones, but by far the most commonly affected are the pelvis, lumbar vertebrae, the sacrum, femora, tibiae and skull. The distribution is usually asymmetrical and may affect only one hemipelvis.

As few as 5% of affected patients have symptoms of *pain* and it is important to exclude other causes of bone pain in people with radiological evidence of the disease. Many of these patients are found by chance at routine radiological examination or after finding a raised alkaline phosphatase level on routine blood screening for something else.

Many patients will present with symptoms due to *nerve entrapment* by the distorted bone, for example sciatica or deafness.

Bony deformity may be the presenting symptom, as in marked bowing of the tibia or enlargement of the skull.

Sometimes the presenting feature is a *fracture* in the affected bone, most commonly in the tibia or femur.

Vascular problems may occur in advanced cases of Paget's disease owing to the greatly increased local blood supply. This may rarely take the form of cardiac failure due to venous shunting producing high output cardiac states. Sometimes advanced disease in the skull or spinal column may have such a great blood supply that 'steal' syndromes occur, especially if the patient has extracranial artery atheroma, and symptoms similar to vertebro-basilar insufficiency with giddiness and nystagmus occur. These patients respond satisfactorily to treatment.

Paget's disease may be severe enough to cause *hypercalcaemia* due to increased bone resorption. This is especially likely to occur if there is immobilization. The hypercalcaemia may cause confusion and nausea and vomiting. The increased calcium excretion in the urine may cause renal stones.

The incidence of *sarcoma* in long-standing Paget's disease has been overestimated in the past and the incidence is probably less than 1% of affected patients.

Investigations and differential diagnosis

The *early lytic phase* of Paget's disease may present difficulties on radiographic examination since it may mimic metastatic neoplasms. As the osteoblastic response becomes predominant the picture grows much clearer and there is a mixture of *lytic and sclerotic areas.* Cortical thickening of the bones then becomes apparent with destruction of the normal trabecula pattern. The disease always starts at one end of the bone and spreads along it. In advanced cases the bowing of the tibiae may be seen with incomplete fissure fractures. Deformity of the base of the skull is known as *platybasia.*

In difficult cases it may be worth requesting a *bone scan* where the lesions show up clearly; this is particularly helpful in lesions in the ribs and scapulae.

Biochemical tests (see Table 3.2) show a very great increase in the *serum alkaline phosphatase* level, which is a measure of the extent of the disease. In patients with disease localized to one or two small bones, the level may be within normal limits. The *blood calcium* level is usually normal unless the patient has been immobolized. The *urinary excretion of hydroxyproline* is raised and is a measure of the collagen breakdown in bone.

Management

The majority of patients have no symptoms and, therefore, require no treatment. There is no evidence that treating asymptomatic patients with drugs such as calcitonin or diphosphonates will alter the extent of the disease or its possible complications, although bone turnover is much reduced by these drugs.

Bone pain may respond satisfactorily to simple analgesics or one of the non-steroidal anti-inflammatory drugs (e.g. indomethacin, ibuprofen, etc).

Patients who have significant symptoms and who do not respond adequately to simple treatment should be considered for long-term treatment with either calcitonin, the diphosphonates or mithramycin. This is especially true for patients who have evidence of a high bone turnover (a considerable elevation of the serum alkaline phosphatase).

Calcitonin has been available for over ten years and is very effective in reducing osteoclastic bone resorption and hence bone turnover. Calcitonin is available in porcine, salmon and human forms and is given by either subcutaneous or intramuscular injection. A typical regime would be to use the salmon preparation (Salcatonin, 'Calsynar' 100 iu daily) for three to six months. Apart from symptomatic monitoring, regular estimations should be made of the alkaline phosphatase level in the serum and, if possible, the urinary excretion of hydroxyproline. Further courses can be given as necessary. The majority of patients respond to this therapy, but in about a quarter the effectiveness will be reduced after a time due to the development of antibodies to the drug. Some patients will become nauseated or flushed with this form of treatment. The nausea is usually controlled with metoclopamide (Maxolon).

If calcitonin treatment fails to control the symptoms or cannot be tolerated, an alternative is the diphosphonate drug, *disodium etidronate* (*EHDP*), in a dose of 5 mg per kg body weight, daily by mouth. This drug inhibits bone resorption and formation. Like calcitonin it should be given in a long course of 3-6 months. It may cause demineralization on bone and produce symptoms similar to osteomalacia. Other side-effects are abdominal discomfort and diarrhoea. It is important to monitor the serum alkaline phosphatase and calcium levels.

If the above regimes are not tolerated or unsuccessful it is possible to use *mithramycin* (Mithracin), a cytotoxic antibiotic which inhibits the transscription of RNA. It has a particular action on osteoclasts and reduces both the alkaline phosphatase level in the serum and the urinary hydroxyproline. It is used intravenously in a dose of 10 μg per kg body weight daily for 5-10 days. It is very much a last resort drug and should only be used for resistant cases as it has a lot of side-effects and causes liver and renal impairment and nausea. Such cases are probably better referred to a specialist physician.

Fractures of the femur and tibia should be treated in the normal way with open reduction and internal fixation, although non-union of such fractures occurs more frequently than in normal subjects. Neurological complications, such as spinal nerve compression, usually respond rapidly to calcitonin treatment, but in rare resistant cases decompression surgery may be indicated.

Malignant disease: primary tumours of bone

Benign tumours of bone in the elderly are extremely rare and are unlikely to be seen in general practice.

Malignant tumours will occasionally be seen. They include:
Osteosarcoma
Chondrosarcoma
Reticulum cell sarcoma
Myeloma

Osteosarcoma usually occurs in patients with Paget's disease in the elderly age group and is said to occur in up to 1% of these patients. The presenting features are bone pain and swelling or sudden fracture. The prognosis is extremely poor and does not appear to be altered by either surgery or radiotherapy. These procedures should be reserved only for the relief of symptoms.

Chondrosarcoma is rarer than osteosarcoma and usually arises in the pelvis, ribs, humerus or femur. It presents as bone swelling which may be painless. Some of these tumours are of low grade malignancy and can be cured by excision.

Reticulum cell sarcoma may arise in any bone. It usually causes very painful bony swelling with local lymphadenopathy. Pathological fractures may occur. Local excision or radiotherapy may give the patient a reasonably good outlook.

These tumours are included for the sake of completeness. The place for their management in general practice will be limited to their recognition and referral to a hospital surgeon or oncologist.

Multiple myeloma is the most frequently seen primary tumour arising from bone. It is a tumour of the plasma cells found in the bone marrow.

Clinical features

About two thirds of patients present with bone pain in the back. Compression fractures are common and make the pain worse. Because of the disturbed immunological function these patients are much more likely to develop infections of the chest and urinary tract. The first symptom may be the development of herpes zoster.

A normochromic normocytic anaemia is present in most patients and weakness and fatigue are common.

Investigations and differential diagnosis

Since the symptoms of myeloma are found in many conditions in the elderly, the diagnosis may easily be missed. A high index of suspicion is required. The haemoglobin level is often around 10 g and the ESR is usually greatly accelerated, often above 100 mm in the first hour. These findings should then lead to investigation of the plasma electrophoresis which shows a dense compact band in the B or Y regions in about three quarters of the patients. Immunoelectrophoresis of the plasma will demonstrate the precise nature of the myeloma. If there is still doubt of the diagnosis a sternal marrow aspiration should be performed which will confirm the diagnosis in over 90% of patients. In distinction to other carcinomas in bone the alkaline phosphatase is normal.

The radiological features of myeloma show small well-defined lytic areas in the bone not surrounded by sclerosis. These are found most frequently in the skull ('pepper pot'), the spine and ribs. The appearances can look like simple osteoporosis.

Management

The prognosis in myeloma is extremely poor, but chemotherapy does offer some chance of remission of the symptoms and some extension of life. The treatment most usually favoured is intermittent courses of high dose prednisolone with melphalan. This should be an in-patient therapy and the patient should be referred to a hospital specialist.

Malignant disease: secondary carcinoma in bone

Secondary malignancy in bone is much more common than the primary variety. Skeletal metastases most commonly arise from primary sites in the:
Bronchus
Prostate

Breast
Thyroid
Kidney

Clinical features

Bone pain and pathological fractures are the usual presenting features. Since there is widespread disease these patients are usually very ill and have general features of weight loss and, often, cachexia. Bony metastases may occur very early in the disease, especially in carcinoma of the breast.

Investigations and differential diagnosis

Most patients have an anaemia and the ESR is often raised to high levels. The serum alkaline phosphatase is usually very high in all secondary bone cancers. In secondary prostatic carcinoma the acid phosphatase is also elevated. Rectal examination does not cause a rise of the acid phosphatase as was thought at one time.

Radiological examination may often give the first clue to the diagnosis. Secondary deposits are usually widespread and show lytic lesions in the majority of cancers, although prostatic secondaries are usually mainly sclerotic. The peripheral bones are very rarely affected and the lesions are most usually seen in the spine, ribs, the pelvis and upper ends of the femur and humerus. The bone cortex is usually involved in secondary cancer whereas it is not in osteoporosis.

Management

The majority of these patients are in a terminal phase of their illness and aggressive treatment of the primary site is rarely indicated, although there have been reports of remarkable remission following treatment of the primary lesion in the kidney, for example. In the case of prostatic tumours, low dose oestrogen therapy (stilboestrol 1 mg tds) may provide good symptomatic relief for a time. The survival rate is not, however, affected by this treatment and the side-effects can be severe in men with cardiovascular disease as there is an increased likelihood of thrombo-embolic disease and fluid retention. In these cases orchidectomy may be preferable.

Some palliation of disseminated breast cancer in the elderly may be achieved by giving drugs such as tamoxifen 10 mg bd which block the oestrogen uptake by tumour cells.

Differentiated tumours of the thyroid often respond quite well to radio-

73

active iodine treatment and referral to a hospital specialist in this condition is essential.

Management should be directed at *supportive therapy* for the patient and his family as well as relief of pain. It is important to make sure that the family fully understand the diagnosis and its likely outcome. It is also much easier if the patient can be made fully aware of the situation. There is often considerable reluctance on the part of the family for either the doctor or themselves to discuss the diagnosis with the patient, but in general this reluctance should be overcome. Even if they are not told, most patients will know that there is something seriously wrong. A decision to withhold the diagnosis from the patient erodes the important relationship between him, the doctor and the family.

Pain relief is essential and must be adequate. Simple analgesics, such as aspirin and paracetamol, may be sufficient if given four-hourly in full doses for some patients. Often morphine derivatives and substitutes will need to be given (e.g. MST tablets and diconal) on a regular basis. Prostaglandin inhibitors (NSAIDs) are often extremely effective in the relief of bone pain.

DISEASES AFFECTING MUSCLES AND JOINTS

This chapter will deal briefly with diseases that affect mobility other than neurological problems. This area considers some diseases that may affect all age groups and constitute the major reasons for absence from work in younger people; in the elderly they pose different, but no less severe, problems.

Rheumatoid arthritis

Rheumatoid arthritis (RA) is a systemic connective tissue disorder which principally affects synovial membranes of joints. The disease also affects peri-articular structures, such as the ligaments and the bones as well as non-articular features which include rheumatoid nodules and circulating antiglobulins (rheumatoid factor).

Clinical features

The problem of RA in an elderly person may be the legacy of disease that started in younger age, since the disease is commonest between the ages of 25 to 55 years. However, RA may appear for the first time in old age.

The acute phase of RA does not differ in presentation whatever the age. Symptoms may be variable, but include acute pain and swelling of any synovial joint, most commonly the proximal interphalangeal, metacarpophalangeal, wrists, metatarsophalangeal and knee joints. Less frequently the elbows, shoulders, ankles and hip joints may be affected. The synovium becomes inflamed, tender and swollen with effusion into the affected joint. The peri-articular structures, such as the ligaments, are also involved leading to joint instability and subluxation or dislocation of the joint. The joint tends to be kept flexed in the position of maximum comfort, resulting in contractures as well as joint deformity. Severe disease will finally result in fibrous or bony ankylosis or secondary degenerative change.

The disease is often symmetrical and produces early morning stiffness, which in the early stages tends to improve as the day passes. Sometimes only one joint is involved. Systemic symptoms also occur and include fever, weight loss and malaise. Rarely other structures such as the pericardium or pleura are involved.

More frequently the features of long standing RA will be found in the elderly. These are the end results of the active process described above and will depend both on the severity of the disease and the results of treatment. The hands and wrists are most frequently troublesome from a pain and functional point of view. Active disease with new inflammation is usually absent and the problems are related to the deformity of the joints. The fingers may be deformed in a number of ways. Chronic flexor tenosynovitis and tendon nodules will produce triggering of the fingers with marked loss of power. Palmar subluxation of the proximal phalanges on the metacarpals will produce the swan neck deformity, other deformities that are often seen are the Z deformity of the thumb and the boutonniere of the fingers. There is usually residual spindling of the fingers through chronic swelling of the proximal interphalangeal joint, and the fingers show marked ulnar deviation. The ulnar styloid may be prominent and tender and be associated with rupture of the extensor tendons, especially the 4th and 5th.

The feet are usually involved but are less troublesome than the hands in most patients. They may be chronically painful and dorsal subluxation of the proximal phalanges exposes the metatarsal heads producing pain on walking. Painful callosities are common.

The knee may be extremely troublesome. The ligaments become lax and the joint surfaces damaged resulting in fixed flexion deformities as well as valgus or varus deformities and an unstable joint. This problem is particularly troublesome with obese patients.

The cervical spine may also be involved and produce root pain especially of the 1st and 2nd cervical nerves, although any may be affected. Changes involve all the synovial joints in the neck and there may be subluxation of the vertebral bodies or the atlanto-axial joint. These deformities may also contribute to vertebro-basilar insufficiency as well as producing painful neck movements and root and cord compression symptoms. Considerable care must be taken with anaesthesia.

Synovial-lined bursae at any site may be chronically involved and produce swellings. The sites most commonly involved are the olecranon, prepatellar, subacromial, trochanteric and popliteal bursae. The popliteal bursa swelling is known as a Baker's cyst; this may occasionally rupture and cause a painful tense swelling in the calf, which may mimic a deep venous thrombosis. An arthrogram will confirm the diagnosis.

Septic arthritis is a serious complication of chronic RA, especially in those patients on steroids. Usually only one joint is involved and becomes acutely painful and swollen during an episode of bacteraemia. There is usually some systemic upset as well, but this is not always so and thus makes the diagnosis more difficult. In this situation both blood and joint cultures must be taken and full antibiotic treatment given immediately. Any acute flare-up of a joint in an old person should suggest this diagnosis.

Bony changes occur secondarily to RA. There may be erosions in the terminal phalanges and all bones in association with affected joints will develop some degree of osteoporosis. The vertebrae may collapse and produce further pain and deformity. The osteoporotic changes are more marked in patients who have been given steroids.

Anaemia is often a feature of the acute phase of the disease, but may also occur in chronic patients as a result of gastrointestinal bleeding from non-steroidal anti-inflammatory drugs (NSAIDS).

Investigations

The diagnosis of rheumatoid arthritis is primarily a clinical one, but certain blood tests are helpful. In the acute phase the ESR will be raised and gives some measure of the degree of activity. Anaemia may be present in the acute phase and is normochromic and normocytic. The rheumatoid factor may not become positive for many weeks after the onset of the disease.

Radiography may be helpful in all phases of RA. In the acute phase there is juxta-articular osteopaenia and bony erosions develop around the affected joint margins, especially in the fingers. Later features seen on X-ray include the deformed joint space and valgus and varus deformities especially of the knees. X-rays of the neck should be taken in attempted flexion and extension and may show the characteristic subluxation of the vertebral bodies and atlanto-axial joint described above.

Differential diagnosis

In the elderly polymyalgia rheumatica is a common and important condition which may sometimes be mistaken for RA. Polymyalgia is a disease affecting muscle and there is no true joint involvement. In this condition either the shoulder or pelvic girdle muscles are involved or both. There is a systemic disturbance and often a fever with a considerably raised ESR (usually greater than 80 mm). The differentiation from RA affecting the cervical spine is important since steroid treatment will make the latter condition worse and cause potentially dangerous cervical root or cord compression symptoms.

Asymmetrical arthritis affecting one or only a few joints can be due to RA but must be differentiated from gout, tuberculosis, septic arthritis and the sero-negative arthritides (psoriasis, ankylosing spondylitis, inflammatory bowel disease and Reiter's syndrome). A careful history and general examination should make the differential diagnosis clear.

Management

The acute phase of RA must be treated with immobilization of the affected joints and anti-inflammatory drugs such as aspirin or one of the newer NSAIDs (e.g. indomethacin (Indocid) 25–50 mg tds, diclofenac (Voltarol) 50 mg tds, etc.). Gold and pencillamine have a place in the active disease state although their effects will take some time to appear. It is important to assess the renal function before using these agents. Steroid treatment can be used for severe cases, but the dosage must be kept to a minimum as the side effects in the elderly may be more disabling than the disease. In very severe cases which do not rapidly respond to the above treatment regimes it is better to admit the patient to hospital for complete rest.

Immobilization of affected joints is best achieved by splinting in the position of function. Sometimes flexion deformities of the joint may occur and the patient should then be referred to a physiotherapy department for serial splinting using plaster of Paris or one of the newer heat malleable plastics. It is important for these splints to be light.

As soon as the acute swelling phase has passed physiotherapy is required to strengthen the muscles around the affected joints. This is especially important if the patient has had to be treated with bed rest. Hydrotherapy pools are very useful as this allows improvement of muscle function without weight bearing.

Occupational therapy also has an important place at this stage of treatment, especially if the small joints of the hands are involved. Occupational therapists are especially trained to assess and rehabilitate functional disability in activities of daily living. They are also in a good position to assess the need for aids, such as large-handled knives and other gadgets that will simplify the work of dressing and cooking. The day hospital concept provides a good milieu for combining physiotherapy and occupational therapy assessment and treatment in the same unit and early referral to such a unit is important.

The chronic inactive phase of rheumatoid arthritis is likely to be the area most commonly encountered in the older patient. The problems that are seen here are products of the results of the severity of the active disease and the efficacy of the treatment given at the time. It is important for the doctor to make an assessment of the degree of pain and disability produced by the damaged joints. The general practitioner is in a unique position to make this assessment since he will see the patient in the home situation and can assess the interaction between the patient's functional disability and the practical problems of his or her home conditions as well as the role that is played by relatives in that situation. The following check list shows the common day activities that need to be considered. The details shown in the list will be beyond the remit of the family doctor, but if there is evidence of any significant disability in these areas help should be sought from an occupational therapist, based in either the community or hospital. Again, referral to the local day hospital will enable rehabilitation to be started. In the meantime it may be necessary to arrange for help to be provided in the home, such as district nurse visits, meals on wheels or home helps. Patients need a lot of help and encouragement, but can be reassured that a great deal can be done to improve and support their situation.

Checklist of disability in arthritics

Personal hygiene
    shaving
    washing hands and face
    combing and brushing hair
    getting to and using the lavatory
    getting into a bath and overall washing
    cutting toenails

Dressing
    overall dressing
    fastening buttons and zips
    putting on shoes and stockings

Within the home
  feeding
  preparing meals
  getting in and out of bed
  housework

Mobility
  moving around the house
  climbing stairs
  mobility outside the house

In the community
  local shopping
  using public transport

Drug treatment of the chronic phase of rheumatoid arthritis should generally be limited to simple analgesics. The place for NSAIDs is limited, since these drugs are really only of benefit in the active phase of the disease and as pain relievers are no more effective than simple analgesics. Similarly local joint injections of steroids are to be deprecated unless there is evidence of joint activity. If misused, these injections can accelerate the destruction of joints.

Checklist for management of rheumatoid arthritis

	Acute Phase	Chronic Phase
Immobilization of affected joints	√	—
Active mobilization of affected joints	—	√
Drugs		
Aspirin	√	⎫ if signs of flare up occur
Non-steroidal anti-inflammatories	√	⎬
Analgesics e.g. paracetamol	—	√
Gold	⎱ For	—
Penicillamine	⎰ resistant	—
Chloroquine	cases	—
Steroids	⎱ For few	—
systemic local injection	selected cases	only for local joint flare up

The role of joint replacement surgery in chronic disability is beyond the scope of this book. However, it is clear that the range and effectiveness of joint replacement has improved greatly in recent years. The classic example is total hip replacement, which now has become a standard operation and has good long-term results, although this is rarely indicated for rheumatoid disease (see osteoarthritis below). Smaller joint replacement is more likely to be considered in RA. The results of knee replacement, usually new semi-constrained arthroplasties, are very encouraging but are not universally available. The indications for consideration for this type of surgery depend on a balance between pain and functional disability. In the elderly there is rarely a place for finger, elbow or shoulder joint replacement. If the general practitioner feels that pain and functional disability are such that knee or hip joint surgery is indicated the best policy is to refer the patient to a physician in geriatric medicine or a rheumatologist in the first instance for assessment. In some areas there are joint clinics staffed by physicians and orthopaedic surgeons for such assessment.

Osteoarthritis

Osteoarthritis (OA) is featured by destruction of the articular cartilage and, subsequently, the bone with osteophyte formation. It is a disease of wear and tear and has a close correlation with ageing. Accelerated destruction of the articular cartilage occurs when there is excessive wearing stress, as in manual workers and some sportsmen. Any joint may be affected, but most commonly the spine, long bones in the legs and the hands.

By the age of 65 years, 80-90% of the population have radiological evidence of osteoarthritis, but significant symptoms of pain and disability only occur in about 20%. As the disease progresses secondary ligamentous laxity occurs and the joints become deformed and unstable. Ultimately the joints become damaged to such an extent that subluxation or fusion of the joints occurs.

Clinical features

Pain is the most serious symptom and this is commonest in the spine, hips and knees. Although the disease often affects the fingers the amount of pain is not usually great. It is often difficult to distinguish osteoarthritis from long standing RA, but this is rather academic since the management is much the same. The pain is worst on movement, but in advanced cases may occur at rest and cause problems with sleeping. OA affecting the lumbar spine may result in nerve root pain which can be very distressing. The radiation of the pain may suggest OA of the hips or knees, and careful clinical examination of all these joints will usually clarify the situation. OA affecting the cervical spine may also cause nerve root involvement and radiate to the shoulders, the arms or the neck and head. Movements of the neck are painful and limited. Osteophyte formation may cause compression of the vertebro-basiliar arteries and produce severe giddiness on neck movement.

Pain from OA of the hip and knee may cause some confusion and the location of the pain may not give an accurate picture of the joint affected; careful examination of all these joints is essential.

Functional disability is the other serious manifestation of OA. The hips and knees are the joints that give rise to the most important functional disability. Walking becomes progressively more difficult and immobility leads to increasing dependence on other people for normal activities of daily living. Climbing stairs and getting out of low chairs may become impossible. The shuffling gait produced by bilateral OA of the hips may lead to an increasing propensity to falls by tripping over loose carpets and wires. OA of the knees may also lead to serious problems with gait and, in addition, may lead to falls when the knee gives way through joint laxity.

OA of the shoulders and elbows is much less common but when it occurs may give rise to considerable pain and functional problems with dressing and performing household tasks.

In advanced cases there may be considerable deformity of the joints, and this is particularly true of the knee joints, which may be either varus or valgum. The mechanical stress produced by these deformities will ultimately lead to problems in other joints, especially the contralateral hip and the lumbar spine.

Effusions within the joints and synovial swellings, such as the Baker's cyst in the popliteal fossa can be demonstrated. A Baker's cyst may rupture and produce symptoms very similar to a deep venous thrombosis in the calf (see above).

Management

The diagnosis is assisted by radiological examination of the affected joints. The assessment of functional disability should be made as for RA (see above).

The management of pain and functional disability are the same as for RA (see above).

The special situation of OA of the spine requires careful assessment. Prolapsed intervertebral discs are not uncommon in the elderly and should be treated by bed rest and, if there is root pain, traction. Epidural injections of long-acting steroids may be very helpful if the pain does not settle in a week or so. Lumbar spondylosis will also be helped by physiotherapy in the form of heat and mobilizing exercises. When these measures fail to produce relief a supportive lumbar corset may be helpful. Many of these patients are considerably overweight and dieting should be part of the general treatment.

Similar approaches should be made in the management of cervical spondylosis. If radicular symptoms or vertebro-basilar insufficiency are troublesome a plastizote collar may be very helpful. For the rare cases where cord compression occurs it will be necessary to seek an urgent neurosurgical opinion.

Crystal synovitis

Gout may occur in old age and is caused by deposition of monosodium urate crystals in the joint. It is commonly precipitated by the administration of diuretic drugs and occasionally it may be caused by blood dyscrasias. There is rarely a family history of gout in the elderly.

The diagnosis of gout is usually easy if there is a sudden onset of acute podagra, but this only occurs in less than one half of the patients. Any joint may be involved, but apart from the first metatarsophalangeal joint the knee is most usually affected. The diagnosis is confirmed by finding a raised serum level of uric acid, and if the knee joint is involved aspiration of the synovial fluid will show the negatively birefringent crystals of monosodium urate.

Pseudogout may also be seen in the elderly and is caused by deposition of calcium pyrophosphate crystals in the joint. These crystals are weakly positively bi-refringent. The knee is the joint most commonly affected and radiological examination may show calcification of the menisci chondrocalcinosis). A similar picture can be seen when the radio-ulnar joint or the symphysis pubis are involved. Hyperparathyroidism and haemochromatosis will also cause chondrocalcinosis and it is therefore important to measure the serum levels of calcium, alkaline phosphatase, phosphate and the iron and iron-binding capacity in all cases.

Management

The management of acute crystal arthropathy is the same whatever its cause. The joint should be rested and a NSAID, such as indomethacin (Indocid) 25–50 mg tds, given by mouth. If the serum uric acid level is found to be high long-term treatment with allopurinol (Zyloric) 300 mg daily should be given to reduce the serum uric acid, the level of which should be monitored. Drugs of the diuretic group should be stopped or, at least, reduced to the minimum. When allopurinol treatment is started it is wise to cover the first month's treatment with a non-steroidal anti-inflammatory drug.

Other arthropathies

Neuropathic arthropathy may occur when there is impairment of pain or joint position sensation. This is most commonly seen in patients with diabetes, especially if they are not well-controlled. Much rarer causes are tabes dorsalis and syringomyelia. The problem may be caused if there have been excessive intra-articular steroid injections. In these situations the joints are painfree and usually greatly disorganized. The knee is most commonly affected and leads to severe impairment of mobility.

Some malignant diseases can involve the joints apart from blood dyscrasias. Carcinoma of the lung may produce hypertrophic osteoarthropathy – clubbing of the fingers and toes and enlargement of the extremities. This is caused by periarticular and periosteal thickening. A similar situation can occur in mesotheliomas of the pleura. The arthropathy may precede the underlying tumour. Myeloma may also cause a polyarthritis resembling RA due to amyloid deposition in the small joints.

Soft tissue lesions

Capsulitis of the shoulder is a common problem in the elderly and may occur spontaneously or after trauma, such as upper limb fractures, hemiplegia and myocardial infarction. This produces an inability to actively elevate the arm and a loss of passive movement of the shoulder joint.

Supraspinatus tendinitis may occur after a fall on the shoulder or excessive exercise of the joint. A full range of passive movement is possible but there is painful active abduction of the arm. Calcific deposits may be seen in the supraspinatus tendon on X-ray.

These conditions can usually be easily treated with physiotherapy, but if this fails to produce relief in a week or so hydrocortisone injection of the joint should be given.

Other soft tissue lesions are common in the elderly and these include plantar fasciitis, tennis elbow (lateral epicondylitis) and golfer's elbow (medial epicondylitis). These conditions are usually easily cured by local injections of hydrocortisone.

STROKES

A stroke is a sudden disturbance of cerebral function of vascular origin causing motor or sensory disability lasting more than 24 hours or leading to death within that time.

The pattern of disability following stroke is very variable although it usually affects one side of the body. The 'sudden' onset means that it occurs over some hours or even less rather than over many days. Stroke is a cerebro-vascular phenomenon, although a similar clinical picture can be produced by other pathologies, such as a cerebral tumour. If the stroke recovers within 24 hours it is referred to as a transient ischaemic attack. A relatively new term has been coined for those strokes that recover completely after 24 hours but within a week – reversible ischaemic neurological deficit (RIND). The importance of differentiating between these three main forms of stroke is that the prognosis for functional recovery and long-term survival is different.

Aetiology

In the elderly stroke is as common as ischaemic heart disease and after the age of 75 it occurs more frequently. To put this into perspective, a new stroke will occur in two per 1000 population per year and in the same population there will be a further five survivors of previous stroke. If the proportion of the population aged 65 years and over is greater than the current norm of 15% (in Great Britain) then the incidence of stroke will be higher.

Strokes are the result of obstruction to blood flow in the brain and are usually associated with widespread arteriosclerosis. The obstruction may be in the main vessels originating from the circle of Willis, usually the middle cerebral artery, or in either the carotid or vertebral arteries. The extent of the infarcted area will be governed by the effectiveness of the collateral circulation available to the affected area through the circle of Willis. Also some 'autoregulation' of cerebral blood flow can be achieved by constriction or dilatation of cerebral arterioles, although this mechanism is not very effective in the old. Autoregulation is related to systemic arterial pressure. At low systemic pressures, when arteriolar dilatation is maximal, any further fall will reduce cerebral blood flow. In chronically hypertensive patients the autoregulatory mechanism is set at a higher level and inappropriate attempts to lower the systemic blood pressure may result in a reduction of cerebral blood flow that would not occur in normal subjects at the same pressure.

Causal factors in stroke in the elderly are not all that clear. Hypertension in younger life results in acceleration of atheroma and a higher incidence of stroke. Smoking in middle-aged people is also associated with a higher incidence of stroke, but this may not be true for elderly smokers.

A raised haematocrit is associated with a higher incidence of stroke, and raised levels of haemoglobin and packed cell volume should be treated by venesection.

Diabetics have a higher incidence of stroke than patients with normal glucose metabolism, and every effort should be made to control blood sugar levels. The mechanism is presumably accelerated atheroma in these patients.

There is no good evidence that obesity and high levels of serum lipids are associated with an increased incidence of stroke in the elderly, but clearly obesity will compromise functional recovery after a stroke.

There is now some evidence that water hardness may confer some protective benefit against both ischaemic heart disease and stroke but the mechanism of this association remains an area of considerable conjecture.

Embolic disease is an important cause of stroke. Emboli can arise from atheromatous plaques in the carotid arteries, from the mural thrombi that may occur after left ventricular infarction and from thrombi in the left atrial appendage associated with mitral valve disease and chronic atrial fibrillation.

Clinical features

Strokes may develop over a matter of minutes or up to a few days, depending on the cause. In general terms haemorrhage from a ruptured cerebral artery and emboli from more distant sources will present an acute episode. Cerebral thrombosis and some embolic phenomena may produce a stroke that develops over a day or two. However, the suddenness of the stroke does not give a very accurate clue to the cause since there is considerable variation in different patients.

The clinical picture of neurological deficit will depend on the particular area of the brain that is compromised. Strokes affecting the cerebral hemispheres are five times as common as those affecting the brain stem.

Sudden onset of stroke due to *cerebral haemorrhage* usually presents with headache, nausea and vomiting and rapid loss of consciousness. The paralysis in these patients may be on both sides of the body if the haemorrhage is extensive. The mortality in this situation is of the order of 80%, but those who survive the acute episode may regain substantial neurological recovery.

Cerebral infarction usually has a gradual onset and a fall in the level of consciousness indicates cerebral oedema. Maintenance of a fully conscious level in the first 48 hours after the onset of stroke indicates a good prognosis for survival – about 85%. If the patient is unconscious for over 48 hours after the onset of the stroke, the mortality rate approaches 100%.

The so-called *stroke in evolution* is often due to carotid artery occlusions. The signs of hemiplegia, speech disorder and a gradually falling level of consciousness may take place over several days. It is important to recognize this syndrome as it may be possible to modify its progress. Many of these patients have a carotid bruit in the early phase of the stroke which disappears when the occlusion is complete.

Subarachnoid haemorrhage has a sudden onset with severe headache and vomiting. Neck stiffness is an early sign and there may initially be no paralysis. The cause is usually rupture of an aneurysm and it is more frequently seen in hypertensive patients. Retinal examination often shows signs of hypertensive retinopathy and sometimes flame-shaped haemorrhages.

Localization of the stroke

Strokes occurring as a result of obstruction to the carotid and middle cerebral artery territory produce a hemiplegia on the contralateral side. Speech may be involved if the left side of the brain is affected, even in apparently left handed people. There are two speech centres in the left hemisphere. Broca's area is in the frontal lobe and is responsible for the initiation of speech; damage to this area produces expressive dysphasia where the correct words cannot be found and sentences tend to be short, poorly formed and lacking in fluency. Wernicke's speech area is in the temporal lobe and is associated with the monitoring and reception of speech. Damage to this area produces a receptive dysphasia where speech retains its fluency but the words tend to be nonsensical and sentences full of mistakes. In practice most lesions produce a mixed picture of expressive and receptive dysphasia.

Strokes in the carotid territory usually involve the sensory as well as the motor area. They may also involve the parietal lobe which affects the ability to calculate (acalculia), constructional ability and perception. These patients, therefore, are often unaware of the affected side, including the visual field. Some of these patients may have no significant muscle paralysis but because of the perceptual problem they are extremely handicapped. Visual loss will also occur if the optic radiation is involved, usually producing a homonymous hemianopia.

Strokes affecting the vertebro-basilar territory produce principally cerebellar dysfunction – giddiness with ataxia and nystagmus. Speech may be dysarthric and there may be long motor tract signs on one side of the body. Any of the cranial nerve nuclei may be involved, the most common symptom being a disorder of eye movement producing diplopia. The visual cortex may also be involved and can rarely produce complete blindness. Survivors of brain stem strokes usually make a good recovery.

Management of strokes in evolution and completed strokes

Whether the stroke is in evolution or completed, there is a limit to the amount of investigation and treatment that can reasonably be performed in the home and the best course is to arrange the patient's immediate admission to hospital. In the past the hospital management of these situations has left a lot to be desired, and the acute general medical admission ward is hardly the place for careful assessment and treatment of what may be an eminently treatable condition.

In recent years a movement has been made for the introduction of stroke units, but the long-term results of such units have been disappointing. Medical or geriatric admission wards should be staffed with doctors, nurses and therapists who are trained and interested in the problem of strokes, and to whom are available the full investigative panoply of district hospitals. Many of these patients will require investigations, such as CT brain scanning, to enable accurate diagnosis of their lesions to be made.

Urgent assessment and treatment of the stroke in evolution is necessary if any significant progress is to be made in limiting the neurological deficit in these patients. Venesection, platelet aggregating modifying drugs, dexamethasone, anticoagulant therapy and emergency arterial surgery may each have a place in the emergency management of these patients but the details of these forms of therapy are beyond the scope of this book.

For the completed stroke physiotherapy is the mainstay of treatment. In addition to the physiotherapist, nurses have an important role to play in early rehabilitation since correct positioning of the patient in the acute phase of a stroke may have a significant beneficial effect on the outcome. Active and passive physiotherapy exercises for the affected side are essential in the acute phases of a stroke. Neglect of the affected side is one of the major causes of slow and inadequate rehabilitation and the prevention of early inappropriate reflex patterns of movement is essential.

Early complications of stroke

The commonest early complication of a stroke is the development of bronchopneumonia. Inability to cough properly, diminished chest expansion and immobility are the chief predisposing factors and nursing care should be directed at minimizing these problems.

Deep venous thrombosis, often later followed by pulmonary embolism, is commonly seen after stroke and is due principally to the effects of bed rest and immobility of the legs. The incidence of this complication on the affected side may be as high as 60% in inadequately managed patients. This can be significantly reduced by proper mobilization and there is some indication for the use of low-dose heparin treatment in highly susceptible subjects. If this complication occurs treatment should be with heparin and supportive leg bandaging.

Post-hospital management of stroke

By the time that the patient is ready to be discharged to his home, a full physical, psychological, speech and social assessment should have been completed. With satisfactory home and social conditions, early discharge from hospital should be encouraged since most patients will greatly benefit from the psychological boost of being at home and will feel that progress is really being made in their rehabilitation. This early discharge will impose considerable strain on the primary health team. However, it should not be necessary for the patient to have achieved full walking or dressing independence in most cases. Prior to hospital discharge it is often useful to make a home assessment visit with the patient and his immediate family. This is usually performed by the hospital occupational therapist and should always involve at least the nurse from the primary health care team. Family counselling is very important and the visible assistance of home nursing visits and home aids where necessary must be made available. The continuation of physiotherapy, occupational therapy and speech therapy is vital at this stage. The best medium for this treatment is the day hospital, where the patient should get as much, and usually more, rehabilitation than he would have got in the ward situation. Results of treatment in properly organized and staffed rehabilitation day hospitals are impressive and go a long way in preventing the high incidence of depression that so often befalls the stroke patient.

Transient ischaemic attacks (TIAs)

Transient ischaemic attacks are, by definition, neurological disabilities caused by vascular lesions which recover completely within 24 hours. The commonest causes are stenosis of either the carotid or vertebro-basilar arteries. Other important causes are micro-emboli from either the carotid arteries or from the heart. These cardiac emboli are usually a result of previous myocardial infarction with development of mural thrombi, or occur in patients with atrial fibrillation and associated mitral valve disease. Periods of asystole, such as are seen in the sick sinus syndrome, may produce a similar clinical picture. Rarer causes include cranial arteritis, in which retinal artery occlusion may occur quite suddenly. If this condition remains undiagnosed and untreated there is a high incidence of cerebral artery thrombosis and completed stroke.

Vertebro-basilar ischaemia ('insufficiency')

These attacks are common in the elderly and are usually caused by stenosis in the vertebro-basilar tree, often associated with spondylosis of the cervical spine. Extension and rotatory movements of the neck will produce pinching of the narrowed vertebral artery and give rise to brain stem ischaemia.

A rarer type of brain stem ischaemia is produced by the subclavian steal syndrome. The pathological basis for this condition is stenosis of the subclavian artery, which results in retrograde flow in the vertebral artery in order to by-pass the stenosis on movements of the arm on that side. This condition accentuates the importance of listening for bruits in the neck in all patients with TIAs and vertebro-basilar insufficiency.

Prevention of stroke

Patients with TIAs require full investigation if a stroke is to be avoided in the future. If extensive atheroma is found in one or other of the common or internal carotid arteries a direct surgical approach to remove the atheromatous plaque should be considered. If the atheroma is widespread surgery is less likely to be effective and a medical approach with anti-platelet treatment is indicated.

If the atheroma is limited to the neck artery of the affected side, carotid endarterectomy should be considered. Complete blockage of the carotid tree would mean that bypass grafting of the vessel is indicated. Recently there has been a move to develop extracranial–intracranial vessel anastomosis, most commonly by linking the superficial temporal branch of the external carotid artery to a viable branch of the middle cerebral artery. In the present state of our experience this sort of operation is reserved for patients who have had a cerebral infarction, who are left with only mild or moderate disability, and in whom complete obstruction of the internal carotid artery on the affected side has been demonstrated.

Vertebro-basilar insufficiency can usually be alleviated by immobilization of the neck in a suitable cervical collar, together with the use of anti-platelet drugs, such as aspirin 300 mg daily and dipyrimadole (Persantin) 100 mg tds. The subclavian steal syndrome can be alleviated by removal of the stenosis in the affected subclavian artery by surgical means.

In younger patients the control of hypertension following stroke poses a difficult clinical management problem. In the presence of other target organ damage assessed by fundoscopic examination, electrocardiography and tests of renal function, gentle reduction of the blood pressure is indicated. For those patients over the age of 75 years it is highly unlikely that reduction of the blood pressure is indicated and it may be positively harmful.

Patients who have cranial arteritis require urgent recognition as immediate treatment of this condition with steroids should prevent further cerebro-vascular episodes.

Despite the lack of evidence implicating diabetes, hyperlipidaemia and smoking in stroke occurrence in the elderly, it is wise to try and ensure good control of blood glucose and fat levels in these patients and to stop them smoking.

Prevention of further stroke in those who have had a completed stroke is problematical, but the authors' practice is to use long-term anti-platelet treatment with aspirin and dipyrimadole.

The management of the patient with long-term disability from stroke

The above comments have concentrated on the management of patients who make significant recovery from stroke. However, even with the best treatment, there will be some survivors of stroke who have significant disability. Some of the advances in medicine in recent years have highlighted the possibilities of creating functional independence in very disabled patients, largely as a result of research into crippling diseases such as multiple sclerosis, rheumatoid arthritis, accidental injuries and amputation of limbs. The elderly hemiplegic patient can often benefit from a similar approach to that used in younger disabled people.

It is important for patients, their relatives and medical personnel to realise the fact that even with a dense hemiplegia full independent life can be possible. For these patients the role of the occupational therapist is vital. Aids such as properly designed calipers can prevent the major dangers of tripping in patients with residual foot drop. Walking aids have now been designed that require expert assessment for the individual patient and are often beyond the scope of the primary health team. Patient-operated micro-switch electronic devices can provide important help to the disabled hemiplegic, either as functional aids or alarm and communication systems.

This is a specialized area and help must be sought from occupational therapists and others. Similarly, for those who for various reasons cannot relearn functional skills to enable independent walking, consideration should be given to creating the environment for independent wheelchair life. Simple aids or modifications to clothing can make all the difference between independence and assisted-dressing. Aids such as a mechanical or electronic hoist in the home may have a place. If we are to maintain the maximum independence and preservation of dignity and status for elderly survivors of stroke consideration must be given to all of the above possibilities.

SUMMARY

Stroke disease is a major cause of death and disability in the elderly. Prevention of this problem, however, starts much earlier in life with the control of smoking, hypertension and hyperlipidaemia.

Transient ischaemic attacks require instant recognition, assessment and treatment.

Stroke in evolution and completed strokes should generally indicate immediate admission to hospital, since the full range of investigations and therapy are not available to most general practitioners in the home surroundings. Early discharge home after a stroke must be encouraged and rehabilitation continued as necessary on an outpatient day hospital basis. Home support, by both personnel and aids, is essential in the short- and long-term management of the stroke patient.

Prevention of further stroke by medical and surgical management should be considered, but accurate guidelines are not currently available and much must depend on the home doctor's assessment of the individual patient.

PARKINSONISM AND TREMOR

Parkinsonism or parkinsonian sydrome is characterised by:
Tremor
Rigidity
Postural imbalance
Dyskinesia

Although paralysis agitans (the shaking palsy) was described as long ago as 1817 by James Parkinson it is now clear that there are many other disorders that may produce a rather similar clinical picture. These include:
Drug-induced parkinsonism

Post-encephalitic parkinsonism
Multi-infarct cerebro-vascular disease

The parkinsonian syndrome is extremely disabling and occurs in about
1.5% of both sexes and all races over the age of 60 years.

Aetiology

The underlying pathological and consequent biochemical abnormality of
Parkinson's disease is not necessarily related to cerebro-vascular disease.
There is a loss of the pigmented neurones in the brainstem, mostly in the
substantia nigra and its connections. The nerve cells in the globus pallidus
are reduced. Cerebral atrophy is also more common in these patients than
one would expect at a similar age.

The substantia nigra projects through the nigro-striatal pathway to the
putamen and the caudate nucleus. The neurotransmitter released at its
terminals is dopamine. Since there is a loss of neurones in the substantia
nigra there is a corresponding reduction in striatal dopamine production.
In addition there is also a reduction in cerebral noradrenaline and sero-
tonin.

Drug-induced parkinsonism is caused by inhibition of dopamine function. This may be by blocking storage mechanisms in pre-synaptic terminals
by such drugs as tetrabenazine or reserpine, or by blocking the receptor
sites as occurs with such drugs as phenothiazines (e.g. chlorpromazine),
butyrophenones (e.g. haloperidol) and substituted benzamides (e.g. metoclopamide).

Clinical features

The onset of Parkinson's disease is usually very insidious and early diagnosis is extremely difficult. Drug-induced parkinsonism usually occurs
within two or three days of starting the drug or after increasing the dose,
and is probably dose-related.

Tremor is usually the presenting symptom. The tremor most usually
affects the upper limbs and is slow (4–6 cycles per second). Characteristically there is a coarse pill-rolling movement of the hands. More rarely the
head and legs may be affected. The tremor is present at rest and disappears
on movement. It is accentuated by emotional stress and alcohol intake.
Although the tremor may cause severe embarrassment it is not usually
functionally disabling.

Rigidity affects both agonist and antagonist muscles equally and is most

92

marked in the neck and proximal limb muscles. It produces a uniform resistance to passive stretch of the 'lead-pipe' variety. When significant tremor is superimposed on the rigidity it becomes 'cogwheel-like'.

Bradykinesia is the most disabling symptom. It is due to the difficulty in initiating both spontaneous and automatic movements. Thus there is a general poverty of movement, such as a masked face, loss of arm-swinging on walking, loss of blinking, soft monotonous speech and micrographia.

Postural abnormalities include the flexed simian posture, festinant gait and the failure to resist a pushing or pulling stress (retropulsion).

Gastro-intestinal symptoms include excessive salivation and dribbling from the mouth. Constipation is frequent and most patients are unable to maintain their body weight. Dysphagia may also cause a problem.

Mental disturbances were not described by Parkinson in his original essay, but many patients exhibit progressively severe and disabling intellectual deterioration and psychiatric symptoms. In the advanced stages of the disease dementia is common. Many of these patients become depressed and have confusional states. Sometimes frankly psychotic symptoms occur, with delusions and hallucinations, as the disease advances.

Complications

The main problem with parkinsonism is the reduction in mobility and the ability to lead an independent life at home. These problems are exacerbated by the development of intellectual impairment and psychiatric symptoms. Relatives progressively find that their supportive efforts become strained and this often leads to a breakdown in the home situation.

As the disease advances the extreme mobility problems and dementia contribute to both chest and urinary tract infections. The commonest cause of death is bronchopneumonia. Although modern treatment has enabled considerable advances to be made in the management of immobility the long term prognosis may not be benefitted, and after ten years about 80% of patients are either severely disabled or dead.

Differential diagnosis

Apart from drug-induced parkinsonism there are a number of rarer diseases that should be considered.

Progressive supranuclear palsy (Steele–Richardson syndrome) is a rare condition where, in addition to many of the features of parkinsonism, there is a supra-nuclear gaze palsy and these patients cannot look downwards. In addition they have axial rigidity and sometimes upper motor neurone signs.

They are often demented. The course is usually rapidly downwards and treatment is of little help.

The Shy-Drager syndrome is another rare condition where, in addition to many of the features of parkinsonism, there is severe postural hypotension, loss of sweating, impotence, urinary and faecal incontinence. Headache may be a problem and there may be cerebellar and upper motor neurone lesion signs. The prognosis in the syndrome, even with treatment, is very poor.

Normal pressure hydrocephalus is characterized by the rapidly developing triad of dementia, spastic ataxic gait and urinary and faecal incontinence. Bradykinesia, festinant gait and tremor may also occur and mimic parkinsonism. If undiagnosed the outlook is very poor, but these patients often respond extremely well to ventriculo-atrial shunting if it is performed early.

Management

The objective of management is to improve mobility and independence by reducing spasticity and bradykinesia. Drug treatment will also have a beneficial effect to some degree on the other associated problems of the parkinsonian patient.

It is important to spend some time counselling both the patient and his relatives. Careful explanation of the nature of the disease is important and an optimistic prognosis should be given since most people believe that Parkinson's disease is a progressively disabling and unalleviable state. With the drugs that we currently have available the outlook for the elderly can be quite good and they may die of some quite unrelated disease before their parkinsonism becomes too much of a problem.

Drug treatment of parkinsonism has been revolutionized by the introduction of laevodopa. Laevodopa administration increases the level of dopamine in the brain and its effect has been increased, and the unwanted effects reduced, by the concurrent use of decarboxylase inhibitor. This agent prevents the metabolism of L-dopa to dopamine outside the brain and allows increased replenishment of cerebral dopamine. There are two forms of decarboxylase inhibitor in common use in combination with L-dopa, benserazide (Madopar) and carbidopa (Sinemet). L-dopa treatment does not influence the underlying pathology of the disease and does not prevent the progresssive brain damage that is characteristic of Parkinson's disease. There is, therefore, no indication to use these agents in mildly affected patients. L-dopa should always be used in conjunction with a decarboxylase inhibitor and the choice of compound is largely a matter of personal preference. The decarboxylase inhibitor allows the use of a much smaller dose of L-dopa and so minimizes the unwanted effects of this drug, which are chiefly nausea, vomiting and postural hypotension.

L-dopa should improve up to 85% of patients with moderate or severe parkinsonism. Its benefit in the control of tremor is not as high as this. In the elderly it is best to start with a small dose, such as Madopar 62.5 (laevodopa 50 mg, bensarazide 12.5 mg) or Sinemet 110 (laevodopa 100 mg, carbidopa 10 mg) both twice daily initially. The dose can be increased in the light of clinical progress by one tablet every three days. Both preparations are made in different strengths (e.g. Madopar 125 and 250; Sinemet Plus and Sinemet 250) to allow gentle titration of the dose in an individual patient. Generally it is wise to divide the daily dose and administer the drug three or four times a day in order to minimize the occurrence of the 'on-off' phenomenon, where the patient gets severe swings from mobility to immobility throughout the day due to fluctuating dopamine levels. This occurs especially after a long period of these drugs or at a late stage of the disease. High dose L-dopa preparations usually induce paroxysmal chorea or dystonia. Oroglossal dyskinesia is probably the most noticeable of these effects and consists of purposeless writhing movements of the mouth. The effects usually occur when the parkinsonian symptoms are at their least noticeable. Many patients will accept these involuntary movements without complaint as their disease appears to them better controlled, but if they cause distress the dose of L-dopa must be slightly reduced.

Although it is reasonable to start with L-dopa therapy for moderate or severe disease in the elderly in order to minimize polypharmacy, for the mild case it is sometimes better to start with anti-cholinergic therapy – especially if sialorrhoea is a major symptom. Orphenadrine (Disipal 50–300 mg daily in divided doses) and benzhexol (Artane 2–30 mg daily) are the most widely used drugs. All these agents may cause problems in the elderly, especially in patients with prostatism, narrow angle glaucoma and dementia, which may prohibit their use. These agents may also cause confusion and intestinal obstruction.

Other drugs are available for the mild elderly case. Amantidine (Symmetrel 100–300 mg daily) can be very helpful to some patients and does not have too many unwanted effects, although it may cause confusion and nausea. If depression is an important feature in these patients, amitriptyline (Tryptizol 50–100 mg daily) may be used with good effect.

In recent years two new agents have been produced which are particularly beneficial when used in conjunction with L-dopa and allow the dose of the latter to be reduced considerably. Bromocriptine (Parlodel 10–140 mg daily in divided doses) acts as a dopamine receptor agonist. It is very helpful when L-dopa is producing side-effects or when there are disabling fluctuations in symptoms during the day. It is essential to start with a small dose (2.5 mg) given after the evening meal, as it may cause marked postural hypotension. The dose is then increased by 2.5 mg daily on alternate days until the desired effect is achieved.

Selegiline hydrochloride (Eldepryl 5–10 mg daily) is a selective Type B monoamine oxidase inhibitor and can be used safely with L-dopa and without dietary tyramine restriction. It potentiates L-dopa and is useful for the patient with laevodopa-induced end-of-dosage deterioration. It may produce nausea, vomiting and dizziness.

Physical therapy is very important in the parkinsonian patient. Outpatient attendance at a day hospital provides a good medium for both patient counselling and for the introduction and monitoring of anti-parkinsonian drugs. Physiotherapy is useful in helping the patient to correct their postural abnormalities, to reduce spasm, to provide walking exercises and to improve upper limb function.

POSTURAL TREMOR

There are numerous causes of postural tremor, of which the most common are:

Benign essential tremor (senile tremor)
Exaggerated physiological tremor
Anxiety
Thyrotoxicosis
Alcohol
Caffeine
Drugs (salbutamol, lithium, sodium valproate)

Benign essential tremor may start at any age, but in the elderly is generally known as senile tremor. It is usually inherited as an autosomal dominant trait and no obvious biochemical or pathological cause has yet been demonstrated. It does not occur at rest and appears in the hands on maintaining posture. It does not worsen on purposeful movement and rarely causes functional disability. Many patients, however, find it very embarrassing. It tends to be slowly progressive. It is helped by alcohol ingestion and, if treatment is necessary, beta-blocking agents such as propanolol (Inderal 30–120 mg daily) are helpful.

SUMMARY

Parkinsonism affects a significant number of elderly people and may cause a great deal of disability. Although it is a progressive disease, with modern treatment it is possible to alleviate many of the disabling symptoms. Patient and family counselling together with careful manipulation of drug control will demand a lot of the general practitioner's time and skill.

INCONTINENCE

Urinary or faecal incontinence is defined as the involuntary or inappropriate voiding or urine of faeces to such an extent that it causes a social or hygenic problem.

Aetiology

At least one quarter of all those over 65 years will suffer from incontinence at some time or other.

The commonest type of incontinence of urine is due to urethral leakage in both men and women. Less common causes of urinary incontinence in women are extra-urethral leakage due to vesico-vaginal and uretero-vaginal fistulae.

Urinary incontinence in women is the most frequently encountered problem in clinical practice and may be due to:

Urinary infection
Incompetence of the urethral sphincter mechanism
Overflow subsequent to excessive bladder distension
Unhibited detrusor activity associated with urgency
Reflex incontinence in the absence of urgency
Generalized physical illness and mental confusion

Urinary incontinence in men is less common and usually due to:

Urinary infection
Neuropathic disorders affecting the detrusor mechanism
Overflow incontinence due to bladder neck obstruction
Post-prostatectomy
Generalized physical illness and mental confusion

Faecal incontinence in both sexes is less common than urinary incontinence, but may be associated with it. The most frequent causes are:

Overflow faecal incontinence due to impaction of faeces in the rectum or sigmoid colon
Weakness of the pelvic floor muscles and/or the external anal sphincter
Severe diarrhoea
Mental confusion

Neurogenic incontinence of both urine and faeces are the commonest and most difficult to treat in the elderly. The management of these problems will be discussed in some detail below. The physical structural disorders that produce incontinence are also very important, especially since they are relatively easy to correct. They can be elucidated by careful history-taking and thorough physical examination. They include:

In Men	*In Women*
Prostatic hypertrophy	Uterine prolapse
Impaction of faeces	Ureterocoele and cystocoele
Urinary infection	Senile vaginitis
Rectal prolapse	Urinary infection
Post prostatectomy	Impaction of faeces
	Rectal prolapse

Management of structural disorders

Many of the structural disorders, such as prostatic hypertrophy, rectal prolapse and, often, significant uterine prolapse are best treated by referral to a surgeon for correction. Minor degrees of uterine prolapse in women can be adequately controlled by insertion of a suitable ring pessary. Senile vaginitis in elderly women can easily be controlled by local oestrogen application which will reverse the atrophy of the stratified squamous epithelium in the vagina, the urethra and the bladder trigone, since these structures are hormone-dependent.

Urinary infections in both men and women are often associated with structural disorders. In addition to a thorough physical examination it is important to send the urine off for culture in all patients with incontinence of urine.

Impaction of faeces frequently gives rise to both urinary and faecal incontinence and may not always be easy to diagnose if the impaction is in the sigmoid and descending colon with an empty rectum. Many of these patients are taking analgesic or psychotropic agents and a small percentage may have myxoedema. Many of our elderly patients have diverticular disease of the colon and have for decades taken a diet low in roughage. Adequate bowel clearance must be ensured and a diet high in roughage introduced. If these steps are inadequate laxative agents, such as lactulose (Duphalac), methylcellulose (Celevac, Cologel) or isphaghula (Fybogel, Metamucil) should be used. Elderly patients often find that diets high in bran are unacceptable but may be able to tolerate commercial preparations of bran, such as 'Fybogel'.

Some patients with faecal impaction may have serious underlying lower bowel malignancy; this situation should certainly be considered if there is a history of recently altered bowel habit. It must also be remembered that ulcerative colitis and Crohn's disease of the large bowel do occur in the elderly. If there is any suspicion of underlying serious pathology in the bowel, sigmoidoscopy and barium enema examination should be undertaken.

Prostatic hypertrophy with obstruction of the bladder neck is a common problem in elderly men. A moderate proportion of these patients will have a malignant prostate gland. The principal early symptoms are a poor stream and frequency of urination by day and, especially, by night. These symptoms may be unreported for some considerable time and quite often the first presenting symptoms are those of incontinence with considerable chronic bladder enlargement. Abdominal examination will show an enlarged bladder, sometimes up to the umbilicus. This may be tender. Rectal examination usually confirms considerable prostatic enlargement, but if the middle lobe is enlarged this may not be easily apparent on digital examination. Apart from the size, the consistency of the prostate gland should be noted, as a hard irregular prostate usually suggests malignancy. Many of these patients have associated urinary tract infection, and a urine specimen should be sent to the laboratory for culture. In chronic cases there may be significant renal failure and the blood urea estimation should be performed. The immediate management of bladder neck obstruction should be by bladder decompression with an indwelling catheter. All these patients should be referred to a urological surgeon for transurethral resection and biopsy of the gland.

If the patient is not fit for surgical treatment of their prostatic enlargement the management is by continuous bladder drainage by means of a silastic catheter into a leg bag. The number of patients who require this form of management is extremely few. Silastic catheters do not require frequent changing and may be left *in situ* for many months since they do not get blocked and do not excessively predispose to urinary tract infection. If the urine should become infected it can usually be dealt with by bladder washouts. Antibiotic treatment given systemically in catheter patients is not generally indicated unless there is significant systemic disturbance. In this situation it is difficult, if not impossible, to sterilize the urine and broad spectrum antibiotic treatment usually only converts the infective organisms into strains resistant to the commonly used oral antibiotics.

Malignant prostatic disease should be treated according to the symptoms.

99

Surgical resection should be undertaken if there is significant bladder neck obstruction. Hormone treatment with small doses of stilboestrol (3 mg daily) should only be used if there are symptomatic secondary deposits in the bones. Newer treatments for symptomatic prostatic carcinomatosis, such as estramustine (Estracyt), are promising but should be managed by hospital specialists at our current state of knowledge.

NEUROGENIC INCONTINENCE

The most frequent cause of incontinence in the elderly is impairment of the neurological mechanisms which control micturition. Micturition is a reflex action mediated by the sacral parasympathetic nerves which innervate the detrusor muscles of the bladder and respond to increasing stretch as the bladder fills. Control of micturition is learnt early in life as higher inhibitory pathways develop which suppress bladder contraction until there is a conscious desire to void urine. The sensation of bladder distension is perceived in the frontal cerebral cortex via fibres originating in the bladder and then synapsing in the spinal cord to pass up to the cortex. Descending fibres from the brain pass down the spinal cord to the sacral region and thence to the bladder. These ascending and descending pathways are subject to various facilitatory and inhibitory influences as they pass the brain stem and the spinal cord. Disruption of these pathways at any level may result in loss of bladder control. In disease affecting the higher cerebral centres the normal inhibition of bladder emptying may be lost; this is termed the uninhibited bladder.

If the purely sensory nerves in the posterior spinal cord are involved and the motor pathway remains intact, there is no perception of bladder distension. The dominant inhibitory influence of the higher centres continues to act and the bladder continues to distend until it overflows with incontinence – the atonic bladder.

The lowest level of bladder control is in the sacral nerves themselves; if these are damaged all central control of bladder function disappears – this is known as the autonomous bladder.

MANAGEMENT

The uninhibited bladder

This is the commonest cause of incontinence in the elderly and is usually associated with widespread cerebral disease, such as multi-infarct or senile dementia. Rarely focal cortical lesions, such as parasagittal meningoma, may produce this abnormality. Although bladder sensation is intact contractions occur suddenly and without warning and the whole of the bladder contents are voided. Sometimes there may be little evidence of focal disease and the bladder emptying may be precipitated by a simple stimulus such as a cough or rising from a chair – the 'unstable bladder'. This can be differentiated from stress incontinence where there is only a small leakage of urine.

However laudable increasing patient mobility may be, it will not get over the problem of the uninhibited bladder since there are only a few seconds of warning before complete bladder emptying. Similarly the provision of bedside commodes or bottles will not prevent this form of incontinence. Absorbent pads will also be insufficient since the whole of the bladder contents are voided. Treatment of the unstable and uninhibited bladder should be aimed at blocking the cholinergic impulses to the detrusor muscle or by direct smooth muscle relaxants. The most useful treatment is with imipramine (Tofranil) which has considerable anticholinergic properties. Drugs such as emepronium bromide (Cetiprin) are often used but are poorly absorbed from the gut and may cause a severe dry mouth with ulceration. Of the smooth muscle relaxants flavoxate (Urispas) is often used but there is little evidence for its efficacy. Sometimes it is helpful to use an adrenergic agonist drug such as ephedrine (Expansyl) which increases urethral sphincter tone.

Reflex neurogenic bladder

Both motor and sensory tracts in the spinal cord may be damaged in traumatic cord section or by multiple sclerosis. Since the bladder fills and empties reflexly there is usually little that can be done to control the situation, although a small proportion of patients can initiate reflex bladder emptying by stimulating the skin also innervated by the sacral nerves. The vast majority of patients, however, have to be catheterized permanently.

Atonic bladder

This type of overflow incontinence is associated with painless bladder distension and incomplete bladder emptying so that there is always some residual urine. Chronic urinary infection is common. Bladder neck obstruction by an enlarged prostate gland must be excluded by cystoscopy. In the absence of structural bladder neck obstruction treatment of the atonic bladder is not very satisfactory. A cholinergic agonist drug such as carbachol may be helpful in stimulating the detrusor muscle. An alternative approach is to block the adrenergic supply to the urethral sphincter by using phenoxybenzamine (Dibenyline) although this may produce troublesome postural hypotension.

Autonomous bladder

This is a rare type of incontinence and is usually caused by a cauda equina lesion or spinal artery occlusion. In addition to incontinence there is sensory loss in the skin around the anus which is also supplied by the sacral nerves. Most of these patients require long-term catheterization, although some men can be managed satisfactorily by means of an appliance.

Appliances and catheters in the management of incontinence

Stress incontinence may be managed satisfactorily by a programme of pelvic floor exercises, though in more severe cases surgical repair may be necessary. However, the majority of these patients can be managed very well by using some form of incontinence pad since the urinary leakage is small. Many types are available, such as sanitary pads which form a gel on contact with urine together with an impregnated deodorant. More satisfactory, however, are 'Kanga Pants' which are well fitting and have a pouch for the insertion of the absorbent pad.

Various urinals have been developed, but these are rarely adequate for incontinent women. Men can sometimes be well managed by means of tubing or sheaths but they must be correctly fitted and not interfered with or else the consequent wetness is just as bad as the incontinence.

For those patients in whom a permanent indwelling catheter is to be used, the self-retaining silastic type is the best. These catheters can be left *in situ* for many weeks and the only indications to change them are either urinary infection or irritation. A proper leg bag should be fitted with a one-way valve to prevent retrograde passage of urine up the catheter.

Management of faecal incontinence

Impaction of faeces causing either faecal or urinary incontinence or both has already been discussed. There remains a small group of patients who persist in being faecally incontinent and in whom no structural cause can be found and remedied. Faecal incontinence can be caused by neurological degeneration such as dementia or cerebrovascular disease analogous to the uninhibited bladder. Some of these patients can be managed by making use of the gastro-colic reflex by sitting them on a lavatory or bedside commode with a gastric stimulant such as tea or coffee in the morning. If such measures fail, it will be necessary to keep the patient constipated by drugs such as codeine phosphate, and to empty the bowel regularly once or twice a week using enemata or suppositories.

THE ELDERLY DISABLED

Although 95% of the elderly are managed in the community and make up a large part of the general practitioner's workload, little thought is usually given to the size of the problem of disability in the community, and even less training is given to medical students and postgraduate doctors in the management of chronic disability. The size of the problem is clearly illustrated in Table 3.3.

Table 3.3 Proportion of persons aged 65 years or more who reported difficulty with common tasks (excluding bedfast persons)
(Source: Shanas *et al.* (1968), *Old People in Three Industrial Societies* (London: Routledge))

Nature of task	Percentage reporting difficulty		
	Britain	*Denmark*	*USA*
Walking up/down stairs	27	37	30
Getting about the house	7	7	6
Washing/bathing	8	9	10
Dressing/putting on shoes	10	12	8
Cutting toenails	33	31	19

Although they are by no means all old, about half a million people are registered as disabled in Britain. One also has to take into account the fact that a significant proportion (29%) of elderly people live alone, often in very unsuitable housing and without the sort of amenities that most younger people take for granted e.g. a telephone, car and refrigerator. The problem is likely to get worse as the proportion of the very elderly rises in the next two decades. It has been shown, for example, that 22% of those in the age group 65–74 years are handicapped physically, but this figure rises to over 37% after the age of 75 years.

The thrust of public opinion and government policy in recent years has been to attempt to keep more old people in the community, thus explicitly moving away from the provision of residential care. This ideological change to community care has coincided with two other major changing factors which make its implementation more hazardous.

Firstly there are the demographic changes that have occurred in the family structure. Few families now have a large number of children and thus the number of potential carers is reduced. In addition, those potential carers are now more likely to be in part-time or full-time work than previously. The number of divorces has also increased which leads to more complicated family patterns. Changing work patterns have led to increased social mobility which has contributed to the erosion of extended family networks. Furthermore, the women in the family used to be the traditional major source of care for the disabled elderly, but more of them are now seeking employment outside the home.

Secondly the role of the state as the major provider of social support services has undergone a change in emphasis. There appears to be a swing in government policy to diminish its role and to look more to the provision of services from the voluntary sector.

Thus the role of the general practitioner in the years ahead will become more complex, his workload will be greater, and his ability to help coordinate supportive agencies will require more skill. In addition to the patients there will be increasing demands on the practitioner's time in helping the carers. This will be especially true of those suffering from dementia. The fact that a recent study has shown that 48% of those with severe dementia had not seen their general practitioner in the three months prior to the study, and that 60% of those with severe dementia had never seen a psychiatrist does suggest, that in some areas at least, community health care is not all that it might be.

How to maximize resources

Elderly patients may be suffering from a combination of physical disabilities. Those who have suffered from rheumatoid arthritis for years and have coped adequately may become disabled from their osteoporosis, osteoarthritis in other joints, a stroke or Parkinson's disease. Any number of these and other physical illnesses may coexist and go to make up the complexity of disease in the elderly. Medical training has encouraged doctors to look at the pathology of disease rather than the practical problems that occur as a result of it. Patients and their carers are much more interested in being able to get to the lavatory in time to avoid incontinence than they are knowing about the details of CT brain scanning after their stroke!

The district nursing service is the general practitioner's mainstay both in keeping abreast of happenings in the home and family, as well as in providing essential nursing treatments in the home and bathing assistance. The integration of the nursing service into practices has improved this vital relationship. Health visitors are often more concerned with home problems at the other end of life, but also play an important role in screening for disease and disability in the elderly. In some areas the employed practice nurses are also increasingly involved in screening and long-term supervision.

Traditionally the relationship between medicine and nursing has always been close, but the same is not true of practitioners in other disciplines, such as therapists, social workers and chiropodists.

Physiotherapy

Physiotherapists are usually hospital based but in some areas there are community physiotherapists as well. They are concerned with joint mobility, muscle power, posture and muscle and ligamentous strains. It is essential to communicate closely with the physiotherapist so that he or she can provide the best treatment for the patient. Patients also need to understand that physiotherapists can only effect improvement with the patient's co-operation and effort. Long continuation with physiotherapy will not be indicated, except in rare circumstances, and endless physiotherapy does not produce endless improvement. Maintenance and further improvement has to be achieved by the patient working with his exercises at home after an initial spell of sessions with the physiotherapist.

The correct posture is essential if joints are not to be damaged in arthritic and muscle disease. This may be a counsel of perfection in patients with strokes and severe scoliosis, but the best possible posture must be maintained. Hence there are certain other measures that patients with mobility problems have to take, however difficult and unpleasant. Weight should be maintained at the minimum possible. Patients should stand as straight as possible and avoid sitting for long periods in chairs. This latter habit is a major source of flexion deformities of the hips and knees which may take weeks of hard work to correct – if it is ever possible. The posture in bed is important for patients with acute flare-ups of arthritis, and after strokes or other disabling illnesses. Patients may find it comfortable to sleep or lie with a pillow under the knees, but in a patient with active arthritic disease this will very rapidly lead to a flexion deformity of the knees. If full extension of the knee is painful in acute arthritis the joint should be injected with a steroid and ice packs applied to relieve the pain. Further resting of the joint can be achieved by means of a lightweight splint, and it is often helpful if the patient can lie on his face for some periods during the day to reduce flexion of the hips and knees.

The redevelopment of muscle power is a major function of physiotherapy in the elderly after strokes and in chronic arthritic conditions. All joints are to a greater or lesser extent supported by adequate muscle tone and if this is lacking the joint becomes unstable – viz. the frequency of dislocation of the shoulder joint on the affected side after a stroke. Faradism is a useful method for getting voluntary muscles to contract, but it must be done in conjunction with subsequent active exercises. These muscle exercises should be isometric. Patients should be taught these exercises for them to do at home.

When asking a physiotherapist to help a patient it is important to have a general idea about what she can do in the way of treatment. Heat treatment may be superficial or deep. *Superficial heat* will reduce the congestion in an inflamed joint by increasing skin vasodilatation. *Deep heat*, given by microwave or shortwave, will increase the intra-articular temperature and will be of help to patients with osteoarthritis, but may well cause a flare-up of a joint actively involved with rheumatoid disease.

Cold treatment with ice packs can be quite painful, but will slow the activity of joint enzymes and reduce inflammation and swelling. Ice packs will allow considerably less painful mobilization of an inflamed joint.

Occupational therapy

The occupational therapist is an important part of the rehabilitation team and is usually based in hospital. However, many local authority social service departments employ occupational therapists for domiciliary work.

The main work of occupational therapists can be divided into four areas. One is the *assessment* of the practical day to day problems encountered by the elderly disabled patient. This assessment cannot be easily undertaken in a short time in the surgery, and must take place over some days, preferably in the patient's home. Because of the shortage of suitable staff the assessment may have to take place in the hospital situation in the first place with a later domiciliary assessment.

The prevention of deformity is another area which the occupational therapist shares with the physiotherapist. The therapist is able to advise the patient on how to protect their joints by removing the major stresses in daily living activities. This will probably involve teaching new techniques and the use of aids.

The provision of splints is best done by the occupational therapist. Splints can be used both to prevent and correct deformity and have to be fitted and supplied on an individual basis. A large range of lightweight, easily mouldable splint materials is now available, and it is helpful if the doctor can clearly identify the specific purpose of the splint, as this will affect the design of the splint and the optimum use of materials.

Compensation for disability by means of the provision of aids and equipment is a special function of the occupational therapist and one that may revolutionize a patient's life. It is essential that the therapist should be involved at all stages in the assessment and choice of aid and that she carefully instruct the individual in its proper use. The private purchase or supply of aids from other people or agencies should be discouraged.

A brief resumé of some of the uses of aids and equipment should illustrate the special skills available through the therapist:

Aids to the personal activities of daily living

The provision of large-handled cutlery will be of great use to those with deformed or weak hands.

The provision of long-handled or electric toothbrushes to encourage good dental and mouth care.

Advising about the suitability of easily fitted and fastened clothing, e.g. the discouragement of back zips and the use of velcro fasteners, long-handled shoe horns and stocking pullers.

Supplying suitable raises to lavatory seats and the installation of properly sited grab rails.

Bath aids: providing suitable grab rails or shower attachments, or advising on the use of bath boards or non-slip mats may make all the difference in enabling a patient to manage on his own or with the aid of an assistant.

Mobility aids

Walking aids: zimmers, gutter frames, rollator and delta frames

Wheelchairs: these may be self-propelled or electric and can be adapted to fit virtually any patient disability and housing design problem

Domestic aids and equipment

Kitchen aids and adaptations: the kitchen is one of the most hazardous places for the disabled and with care a great deal can be done to make it safe. Correctly heightened sinks and cookers, modified utensils and the use of a perching stool are just some of the very many ideas that are the special expertise of the therapist.

Speech therapy

Speech therapists are, unfortunately, an all too rare commodity for the elderly. Most are going to be hospital-based. They must be used for patients with any speech problems, after a stroke for example. It is very important to make the referral as soon as possible.

Chiropody

Adequate foot care is absolutely essential if the elderly are to be maintained comfortably and safely at home. Although the nurses can deal with quite a lot of minor procedures in foot care, it is surprising how often the foot and footware are neglected. The services of an interested chiropodist are invaluable.

Social workers and community services

Local authorities in Britain are charged with providing a wide range of community services to the elderly and the key to these is the social worker. The range should include:

The provision of meals, either at home or at a luncheon club or day centre.

Practical assistance at home through the home help service.

Arranging for home adaptations to be carried out, usually through the services of the domiciliary occupational therapist.

Assistance in providing home amenities and recreational facilities, e.g. radio, TV, books etc.

The provision of transport facilities to leisure centres and clubs.

The provision of a holiday relief scheme, usually in residential homes run by the local authority.

The installation of telephones and alarm systems.

Social workers are based in both the community and the hospital, and help to bridge this often difficult gap. They are trained to help patients and their families to cope with personal and emotional problems that arise out of disease and disability. They can also provide advice and referral to the relevant resources. They are the key to the range of local authority services and can also help with approaches to other agencies, for example the Red

Cross and the WRVS for the loaning of equipment for temporary periods. They can also help with housing through the local housing department. In addition a social worker can help patients and their families to understand the complexity of the claims and benefits that are allowable and provided by the DHSS.

Individual social workers are increasingly being attached to, or liaising with, primary health teams. This is a development to be welcomed and is a step further towards a truly comprehensive community care team.

The use of the day hospital

Many areas now have a day hospital for the physically disabled elderly. If these are functioning correctly they should be able to provide an excellent short-term rehabilitation service for those in the community. Under one roof there should be the whole complement of the rehabilitation team, including doctors, nurses, physiotherapists, occupational therapists, speech therapists and chiropodists, together with an attendant social worker. The general practitioner should have immediate access to such a unit – if you haven't you should complain!

The day hospital should be able to perform as good or better rehabilitation as can be provided by a hospital ward with the added great advantage that the patient can remain in his own home environment. Day hospitals are tiring for disabled people and it is not often necessary or advisable to send the patient there more than three or four times a week. Unfortunately many day hospitals function as a social support centre and this is a tendency which must be actively discouraged. The function of a day hospital must be for short-term rehabilitation and if it is long-term social support that is required then the patient should be able to go to a day centre or luncheon club. When they function properly day hospitals can do a very fine community job. In addition they should prevent the need for some people ever to go into hospital and they certainly shorten people's lengths of stay in the hospital environment. They also provide that rare commodity: the bridge between those who work in the community and those in the hospital. One of the authors has now opened seven day hospitals with a maximum size of 20 places per day, each taking 300–400 new patients per year, and most of them have a general practitioner on the staff.

It has to be admitted that the above comments may be a counsel of perfection, but in some areas of the country all these services are available. If we are to manage our old people in the community with safety, comfort and dignity then the full panoply of rehabilitation and support services must be made available, if necessary seven days a week. It is important for the general practitioner to know what services can be tapped and how they can be manipulated. If hospital-based therapy or day hospital facilities do not have an open access, if twilight nursing and sitting services are not available, if the local authority has not heard of home care assistants or the housing department does not provide adequate sheltered housing, then every effort should be made to get these facilities improved or changed. In the areas where all these things are available the quality of care that the general practitioner can provide for his patients is high indeed.

PAIN RELIEF

The management of pain may pose considerable problems in some elderly people. Pain is often a very difficult sensation to quantify objectively. Short-term pain presents few problems if the cause is diagnosed and treated effectively, but if this is not done it may become intractable. Pain caused by central nervous system lesions is usually the most difficult pain to treat effectively, perhaps because the mechanism for the production of pain is so poorly understood.

Peripheral nerve lesions

Entrapment syndromes

The carpal tunnel syndrome is the commonest entrapment syndrome in the elderly and should be easily diagnosed. Sometimes it may be mistaken for a cervical root lesion from spondylosis in the neck. Most chronic pain after decompression of the entrapped nerve disappears completely, but the exception is *ulnar nerve compression* in which the nerve may be further damaged by ischaemia during transposition at the elbow.

Post-herpetic neuralgia

This may present serious and intractable pain in the elderly and seems to become more of a problem as people grow older. If the patients are treated at the onset of the virus infection with idoxuridine, 40% solution in dimethylsulphoxide, there is good evidence that the likelihood of post-herpetic pain will be reduced. Unfortunately acyclovir does not appear to have any beneficial effect on the development of neuralgia, although it is highly effective against the herpes virus.

Trigeminal neuralgia

This is principally a disease of old people, although fortunately not very common in our experience.

Painful peripheral neuropathies

The commonest causes of painful peripheral neuropathy are *diabetic* and *alcoholic* neuropathy.

Phantom limb and amputation stump pain

Unfortunately a number of patients develop long-term problems after amputation. There appears to be no obvious cause for phantom limb pain, but stump pain is due to peripheral nerve injury and occurs especially if the above-knee stump is too short.

Management of peripheral nerve injury pain

Simple analgesia with aspirin or paracetamol rarely helps this type of pain and the stronger analgesics, such as dihydrocodeine and pentazocine, are not much better.

Transcutaneous nerve stimulation (*TENS*) may be helpful in all these situations and is worth trying. TENS is a non-invasive therapy where a pulsed electrical current is applied through electrodes across the skin. The modern generators are small and portable. The aim of treatment is selectively to stimulate afferent nerve fibres in an attempt to modulate the transmission of pain signals. In a small number of patients the pain may initially be made worse, but the main disadvantage is skin irritation beneath or around the electrodes. This form of treatment should not be used in patients with cardiac pacemakers or over skin that is broken or anaesthetic.

Before proceeding to invasive forms of therapy for chronic pain, there are other physical therapies that can be tried. *Ice packs* and *vibration* may help postherpetic neuralgia. If physical therapies fail, *drug treatments* with carbamazepine (Tegretol), either with or without an antidepressant drug, should be tried for all types of nerve pain. Great care should be taken with the dosage of carbamazepine in the elderly. The starting dose should be 50 mg tds increasing gradually up to a maximum of 600–800 mg per day in divided doses. Despite careful treatment with this drug some patients are unable to tolerate it due to the nausea, drowsiness and ataxia that it may produce. It is also worth trying the effect of phenytoin (Epanutin) in patients with painful peripheral neuropathies caused by alcohol and diabetes.

Local anaesthetic nerve block is worth trying in post-herpetic neuralgia and in trigeminal neuralgia. If this approach produces satisfactory results the patient can be referred for more permanent nerve blocking with cryoanalgesia, or thermocoagulation of the ganglion in trigeminal neuralgia.

The above approaches should solve a lot of the problems of chronic pain, but there are some patients who will not be relieved by these measures. In this situation acupuncture may help or, alternatively, the patient may be referred to the local pain clinic. It is essential to try and make sure that the diagnosis is certain, but even if it is not, the patient will require some relief immediately. The need for periodic diagnostic review, however, is important.

Thalamic pain

Thalamic pain is caused by infarction of the contralateral thalamus. The pain in this condition is severe, burning or crushing and intractable. The pain may be accompanied by hyperaesthesia. Unfortunately the pain rarely improves with time unless treatment is instituted. This consists of a combination of carbamazepine with an antidepressant drug such as amitriptyline (Tryptizol). Sometimes TENS may be used with good effect. If these measures fail to produce relief the patient should be referred for sympathetic nerve block to the pain clinic.

Back pain

A long discussion of the many causes and treatments for chronic back pain is inappropriate here. A great deal of backache in the elderly, especially women, is caused by osteoporotic collapse of spinal vertebrae. In a proportion of these patients there is associated osteomalacia, which is part of the bone disease of ageing. This is discussed in more detail on pp. 61–68. Prevention is obviously the best treatment, but in those unfortunates who suffer, simple analgesia should be tried first. The addition of vitamin D and calcium supplements is indicated if there is evidence of osteomalacia. In resistant cases it may be worth trying the effect of sodium fluoride 50 mg daily, which will harden the bones by causing fluorosis. Heat treatment to the affected area may also be of help. External spinal supports may also be used for osteoporotic collapse, but these tend to worsen the local osteoporosis. Androgenic steroids are useless and should not be used.

Osteoarthritic and *spondylitic* spinal disease should also be treated with simple analgesia and spinal supports where necessary. Non-steroidal anti-inflammatory drugs are often used in these conditions, but there is little evidence that they are any more effective than properly administered analgesics, and in a significant number of people they will cause gastro-intestinal bleeding.

Degenerative disease of the spinal facet joints (*facet joint syndrome*) is a common cause of backache. A useful diagnostic test is to infiltrate the affected joint with local anaesthetic which will produce immediate alleviation of the pain. If the pain then recurs the patient should be referred to the pain clinic for coagulation of the articular branch of the posterior root.

Fibrositis, or *myofascial syndrome*, is an ill-defined back pain, but it may be helped by local anaesthetic infiltration of the trigger points.

Malignant disease

About one half of patients with advanced malignant disease will suffer intractable pain. Localized pain, especially in the spine, may be very effectively treated with local radiotherapy. For more diffuse pain radiotherapy is contra-indicated and adequate analgesia must be given. For generalized back pain in secondary deposits from a prostatic carcinoma low dose oestrogens should be given, for example stilboestrol 1 mg tds. For other cancers with spinal metastases corticosteroids may be helpful, especially if there is associated hypercalcaemia.

For severe pain in the terminally ill nerve blocks may be indicated and this will entail referral to the pain clinic. Otherwise opiates may be indicated. It is always best if this treatment can be given orally rather than by injection. MST tablets are ideal for this purpose and can be given twice a day in increasing and adequate dosage. Oral pethidine and cocaine are probably better not used. The oral opiates, other than MST, have a very short effective relief span and have to be given every three or four hours, which means waking the patient at night.

The management of pain relief in terminal care is a skilled and time-consuming procedure and every doctor has to develop his own particular approach to the matter. What is certain is that pain relief is so much more effective if the general support is good. This will almost certainly mean involving the local hospice care team and will entail frequent visits from the doctor. In this way the patient and relatives will feel well-supported and pain relief can be accurately monitored. It is important to watch out for other side-effects of the cancer, such as itching, loneliness and depression, and to treat these accordingly. The analgesic drugs themselves are likely to produce unwanted effects such as constipation and nausea. Perhaps surprisingly, the patient may not volunteer these symptoms and he or she should be directly questioned about them. Most respond very satisfactorily to the appropriate laxatives and anti-emetics. Skilled and sensitive nursing care is vital at this time. Attention to mouth infections, stoma care and pressure sores will all help to make the patient more comfortable and the rest of his or her life more tolerable.

Full and frank discussion and explanation of the situation are important for both patient and relatives. This open approach certainly makes the management easier for the care staff when the end approaches. At this stage further investigations, by blood sampling or X-ray, are usually unnecessary. Needless tests should not be performed unless there is real expectation that, by doing them, revised management will lead to an improved quality of life.

The authors have the impression that there are still too many patients admitted to an institution for their last days. Certainly the wider availability of the hospice care system has enabled more people to spend their last days in the security and comfort of their own home surrounded by their family. It is better to withhold injectable analgesics until the last possible moment since their administration increases the strain on the nursing services and is more unpleasant for the patient. It is at times like this that the whole concept of the primary care team is tested to the limit. Certainly it is not until this final stage that the doctor will know whether he has managed the case well but, if he has, it will make the management of the relatives' bereavement much easier.

ANAEMIA

Anaemia is defined as a haemoglobin level of less than 12 g/100 ml.

Aetiology

Anaemia occurs in 10% of men and 15% of women over the age of 65 years. It has been thought in the past that haemoglobin levels below this range are a normal accompaniment of ageing, but this is not so. There are virtually no specific ageing changes in the blood apart from an increasing acceleration of the ESR, which is probably due to the relative fall of albumin and a rise in globulin values in old age.

Haemolytic anaemias and disorders of haemostasis are not substantially different in the older age group and will not be further discussed.

The high frequency of anaemia in the old is due to the following:

Hypochromic microcytic anaemia:	iron deficiency
Megaloblastic anaemia:	vitamin B_{12} deficiency
	folic acid deficiency
Myeloproliferative syndrome:	polycythaemia rubra vera
	myeloid leukaemia
	myelosclerosis
Leukaemias:	acute and chronic myeloid
	acute and chronic lymphatic
Myeloma:	see pp. 71–2
Bone marow suppression	uraemia
	severe infections
	rheumatoid arthritis
	secondary carcinoma
	myxoedema

Clinical features

The symptoms of anaemia are generally more marked in the elderly than in the young.

Lethargy, weakness, tiredness and dizziness are often found, even in mild anaemia.

With more severe degrees of anaemia *cardiac failure* may develop.

Confusion is often found in megaloblastic anaemia.

Pallor is often difficult to assess in the elderly. There may be associated *angular stomatitis* or *koilonychia* in chronic iron deficiency associated with dietary malnutrition.

Atrophic gastritis may occur in vitamin B_{12} deficiency.

Aortic systolic flow murmurs are often heard in anaemias of all types.

General investigations and differential diagnosis

The results of various investigations will be discussed under the headings of the different types of anaemia.

All patients suspected of anaemia should have a *blood count* performed together with examination of the *peripheral blood smear*.

Since many anaemias in the elderly are mixed, it is useful to estimate the *levels in the serum of iron, B_{12} and folate*.

Some macrocytic anaemias are due to liver disease or alcoholism and it will be necessary to perform the liver function tests, including the GT level. Although myxoedema usually is associated with a normocytic, slightly hypochromic anaemia, it may present with macrocytosis and in these patients a *serum level of T4 and TSH* should be estimated.

Normochromic, normocytic anaemias are usually due to chronic renal failure and rheumatoid arthritis and the *urea and electrolytes and rheumatoid factor* should be measured. A mild normochromic anaemia may occur in polymyalgia rheumatica and cranial arteritis, but this rapidly responds to steroid treatment.

In some patients the diagnosis may still be unclear and then it is necessary to refer the patient to the local pathology laboratory for *sternal marrow examination*.

Hypochromic, microcytic anaemia

Iron deficiency
This is the most commonly found anaemia and accounts for about one half of all cases.

The major cause of iron deficiency anaemia is blood loss, usually from the gastro-intestinal tract.

Hiatus hernia, diverticulitis, large bowel cancer and haemorrhoids are common in the elderly and may present for the first time with anaemia. Careful clinical examination, including a digital rectal examination, is essential. Most of these patients will need to be referred to a specialist for gastro-duodenal endoscopy. In expert hands this should be performed before a barium meal examination is ordered. If large bowel bleeding is suspected the first examination requested should be a barium enema, if necessary followed by colonic endoscopy. The incidence of bowel pathology in these patients is so high that every effort should be made to pursue full investigation if the patient is otherwise fit and well.

Blood loss from the gastro-intestinal tract often occurs with the use of non-steroidal anti-inflammatory drugs; aspirin and indomethacin are, perhaps, the commonest offenders, but all these drugs may cause gastro-intestinal bleeding. All these patients require gastro-duodenal endoscopy and follow-up with examination of the faeces for occult blood. In some cases the bleeding may be both acute and severe and may necessitate immediate admission to hospital.

Iron deficiency may also occur with chronic dietary lack. Many old people either dislike or cannot afford iron-rich foods, such as meat and fresh vegetables. Similarly patients who have had a partial gastrectomy will find that iron-containing foods are indigestible and will avoid them. Malabsorption of iron is less of a problem unless there has been extensive small bowel resection.

Management
Acute or severe gastro-intestinal bleeding will require admission of the patient to hospital.

In less severe and chronic cases of iron-deficiency investigation and treatment can be carried out from the home. Dietary deficiency should be corrected by careful explanation to the patient and his family. Supplemental oral iron should be given, either as ferrous sulphate 200 mg tds, or as in one of the slow-release preparations, such as Feospan 1–2 capsules daily. Most patients can tolerate this treatment and will respond satisfactorily. If oral iron treatment causes problems, such as diarrhoea or indigestion, it may be necessary to give it by intramuscular injection, e.g. iron sorbitol citrate (Jectofer) 2 ml daily for about 10 days until the iron stores are repleted.

The management of gastro-intestinal bleeding will depend on the cause that is found by investigation. Obviously if it is caused by non-steroidal anti-inflammatory drugs these should be avoided in the future. Bleeding piles can often be treated by injection of a sclerosing agent, but the other bowel pathologies will often require surgical treatment in hospital.

Causes of treatment failure include the continued occurrence of blood loss and non-compliance with iron treatment or dietary advice.

Further causes of treatment failure include the failure to recognise co-existent anaemias, such as those due to B_{12}, folic acid or thyroid deficiency. In rare cases there may be an associated pyridoxine deficiency.

Macrocytic and megaloblastic anaemias

These are the second commonest anaemias in the elderly and are due usually to vitamin B_{12} or folic acid deficiency. Both of these subtances are stored in the liver, are intimately involved in DNA synthesis, and are vital to normal haemotopoiesis.

Pernicious anaemia
This is due to a deficiency of vitamin B_{12}. This vitamin is present in meat, some seafoods, eggs and milk. It is absorbed in the terminal part of the ileum provided that there are adequate amounts of intrinsic factor produced by the parietal cells in the stomach. Because of its wide availability in foodstuffs, pernicious anaemia is rarely due to a dietary cause, except in vegetarians and food faddists. The usual cause of deficiency is gastric disease or resection or disease of the terminal ileum, for example Crohn's disease or blockage of the lymphatic drainage in the area.

Investigation
The blood picture shows a macrocytosis and raised MCV. The haemoglobin

may have fallen to very low levels as the onset of the disease is very insidious and values of 6 gm/100 ml or less are common.

With severe degrees of deficiency there may be a pancytopaenia with reduction of both white cell and platelet counts.

It is important to send off blood for estimation of the B_{12} and folate levels before any treatment is started. The same applies to sternal marrow examination which may be performed in difficult cases.

Many patients with pernicious anaemia have achlorhydria and antibodies to gastric parietal cells and thyroglobulins.

Management
Once the diagnosis has been made and the blood levels have been sent to the laboratory long-term treatment with vitamin B_{12} replacement should start. The dose should be given daily for the first week and thereafter every eight to ten weeks. A convenient preparation is hydroxocobalamin (Neo-Cytamen) 1000 μg by intramuscular injection. It is wise to check the reticulocyte count in the peripheral blood on the seventh and ninth days after the first injection to make sure that there is satisfactory bone marrow response. The degree of reticulocytosis will be inversely related to the original haemoglobin value. Since treatment has to be given for the rest of life every confirmatory piece of evidence for the correct diagnosis is important.

Folic acid deficiency
Folic acid deficiency produces a macrocytic megaloblastic anaemia indistinguishable from pernicious anaemia. Folic acid is found in many foods, especially green vegetables, liver and kidney. It is absorbed in the jejunum. Unlike pernicious anaemia the main causes of this deficiency are dietary. This is partly due to the fact that old people dislike or cannot afford these foods. This is especially true if they have had previous gastric resection since most folate-rich foods are bulky and indigestible. Malabsorption from the jejunum is unusual. Folate deficiency may be caused by certain drugs, notably phenytoin, phenobarbitone and some cytotoxic agents. These drugs interfere with folic acid metabolism. Liver disease may cause folic acid deficiency. Some malignant and inflammatory conditions may increase the demands for body folate and thus cause a relative deficiency.

Investigations
The same comments apply as for pernicious anaemia. The serum folate level will be low.

Management
Long-term treatment should be commenced with folic acid supplements and general dietary advice about folate-rich foods. The initial dose of folic acid

is 5 mg tds for two to three months and thereafter 5 mg daily. Even with dietary modification patients on anticonvulsants may require folic acid supplements.

Other causes of macrocytic anaemia include liver disease and chronic alcoholism as a result of interference with both folic acid and vitamin B_{12} metabolism. *Scurvy* may still be seen in patients with the Diogenes syndrome (qv) who are subject to chronic malnutrition even in highly civilized societies. Deficiency of ascorbic acid (vitamin C) interferes with haematopoiesis and may present with either a normocytic or macrocytic anaemia.

Normocytic, normochromic anaemia

These anaemias are rarely severe and the haemoglobin value is usually between 9–10 g/100 ml. The most frequent cause is uraemia due to chronic renal failure. A similar situation may be found in patients with long-standing rheumatoid arthritis. Polymyalgia rheumatica and cranial arteritis may be associated with a mild anaemia of this type, which responds rapidly to steroid treatment. Malignant diseases and some chronic infective conditions may also be associated with normocytic anaemia.

Table 3.4 The investigation of common anaemias (from Martin, *Problems in Geriatric Medicine*, p. 172 (Lancaster: MTP Press))

Investigation	Iron deficiency	Pernicious anaemia	Folic acid deficiency
Haemoglobin	7–11 g/100 ml	5–10 g/100 ml	5–10 g/100 ml
MCHC	Low	Normal	Normal
MCV	Normal	High	High
Peripheral blood	Hypochromic, microcytic	Macrocytic	Macrocytic
Serum iron	Low	Normal	Normal
Iron binding capacity	Increased	Normal	Normal
Iron saturation	Low	Normal	Normal
Serum B_{12}	Normal	Low	Normal
Serum folate	Normal	Normal	Low
Marrow sample indicated	No	Sometimes	Sometimes
Antibodies to thyroglobulin	Absent	Usually present	Absent

The myeloproliferative syndrome

This syndrome consists of polycythaemia rubra vera, acute and chronic myeloid leukaemia, essential thrombocytosis and myelofibrosis. Any one of these conditions may occur singly in a patient but sometimes there is a transition between one and another.

Polycythaemia

Polycythaemia in the elderly is most commonly secondary to chronic lung disease. It may also occur in some tumours, especially hypernephroma. The importance of secondary polycythaemia is the fact that it rarely requires treatment and is not part of the myeloproliferative syndrome.

Polycythaemia rubra vera is a chronic condition more frequently seen in men than in women. There is an increase in the production of red cells resulting in a greater red cell mass. There is an increase in the blood viscosity predisposing to an increased incidence of peripheral vascular obstruction and transient ischaemic attacks. Conversely there may be a haemorrhagic tendency. Patients may complain of tiredness, shortness of breath and headaches. Physical signs include a high colour and an enlarged spleen in about two thirds of patients. The spleen is not enlarged in secondary polycythaemia. Laboratory tests in the differential diagnosis of primary and secondary polycythaemia are summarized in Table 3.5.

Management

Polycythaemia rubra vera should be treated by repeated venesections when

Table 3.5 Differential diagnosis of primary and secondary polycythaemia (from Martin, *Problems in Practice*, p. 173 (Lancaster: MTP Press))

Investigation	Polycythaemia rubra vera	Secondary polycythaemia
Haemoglobin above 19 g/100 ml	Yes	Yes
Packed cell volume > 54%	Yes	Yes
White blood cells and platelets increased	Yes	No
Leucocyte alkaline phosphatase raised	Yes	No
Serum B_{12} raised	Yes	No
Arterial PO_2	Normal	Low
Arterial PCO_2	Normal	Raised
Spleen	Enlarged in 2/3 of patients	Not enlarged

the packed cell volume reaches 54%. This procedure can perfectly well be managed in the community. More permanent treatment can be provided by the administration of radioactive phosphorus (^{32}P) which will require referral to a radiotherapy department. The effects of this treatment will not be fully apparent for about six weeks and in the meantime further venesection may be required. Repeated venesections will deplete the iron stores and supplemental iron may have to be given.

Secondary polycythaemia normally requires no treatment, except in the emergency situation where a patient with severe chronic obstructive airways disease and heart failure fails to respond to conventional treatment. In these rare situations venesection may be life-saving.

Myelofibrosis (myelosclerosis)

Myelofibrosis may occur *de novo* or be secondary to polycythaemia rubra vera or chronic myeloid leukaemia. In this condition the bone marrow becomes infiltrated with fibroblasts and produces a pancytopaenia. Secondary haematopoeisis then occurs in the liver and spleen, and these organs may be greatly enlarged. Progressive anaemia occurs and with it a greatly reduced ability to respond to infections. Sometimes the presenting feature may be left hypochondrial pain due to infarction of the enlarged spleen. In this situation there is further enlargement of the spleen, which is acutely tender. There is also an associated fever.

Management

The diagnosis of myelofibrosis is suspected by the finding of a pancytopaenia. Confirmation is then made by arranging for an out-patient appointment for a sternal marrow puncture. The bone marrow is aspirated with great difficulty and microscopical examination shows fibroblast infiltration with corresponding reduction in the red and white cell and platelet precursors.

There is no effective treatment for myelosclerosis. Anaemia should be treated symptomatically with fresh blood transfusions. Infections should be treated early with bacteriocidal antibiotics. Ultimately the patient will die of overwhelming infection or haemorrhage.

Essential thrombocythaemia

This is a rare condition that may sometimes be seen in old men. There is an overproduction of platelets, which do not function normally and thus result in bleeding tendency.

The platelet count is high in the peripheral blood, and bone marrow examination shows an increase in the megakaryocytes. This condition can

121

be managed on a short-term basis by giving busulphan (Myleran), followed up by injection of radioactive phosphorus by a radiotherapist.

Leukaemias

Chronic myeloid leukaemia (CML)

This condition is not common in elderly people and more often is seen in the middle-aged. It is part of the myeloproliferative syndrome and may be secondary to polycythaemia rubra vera. It may progress to myelofibrosis.

Patients with CML usually present with symptoms of anaemia and recurrent infections. Occasionally splenic pain may occur as the presenting feature.

The diagnosis is suspected from the peripheral blood count, which shows a massive increase in the number of granulocytes and anaemia. A sternal marrow puncture should be arranged, which will show a great increase in the granulocyte precursors together with normal mature granulocytes. The Philadephia chromosome is usually present.

Management

The diagnosis is easily made, but treatment is far from satisfactory. Most patients survive around four years from the time of diagnosis. Busulphan (Myleran) in initial doses of up to 4 mg daily will reduce the white cell proliferation, but does not appear to improve the life-expectancy. It should therefore be reserved for severe cases. As with all chemotherapy for blood disorders, treatment may cause an increase in the serum uric acid content and secondary gout. Larger doses will result in complete bone marrow suppression and a reduced maintenance dose of 0.5–1.0 mg daily should be achieved as soon as a peripheral blood response is seen.

In a few patients the massive enlargement of the spleen may cause severe symptoms, and in these splenectomy may have to be considered.

Chronic lymphatic leukaemia is principally a disease of the aged. It is caused by a tumour of the lymphatic series precursors.

This tends to be a benign condition and is usually diagnosed when a peripheral blood count is done for other reasons. Alternatively patients may present with symptoms of anaemia or with glandular enlargement. Clinically there is usually widespread glandular enlargement and the liver and spleen are usually slightly or moderately enlarged.

The anaemia is usually of mild degree with the haemoglobin value in the region of 10–12 g/100 ml. The white count in the peripheral blood shows considerable increase in the lymphocytes, usually in the range of 30 000–80 000, but occasionally up to 300 000 cells.

Management

Since the majority of patients with chronic lymphatic leukaemia run a very benign course, treatment is rarely necessary and it is sufficient to perform routine peripheral blood counts every three to four months. In patients who develop significant anaemia, or in whom the white blood count rises to excessively high levels (above 150 000), a short course of chlorambucil (Leukeran) 0.2 mg per kg bodyweight orally for up to six weeks will usually reduce the white count to reasonable levels. Other signs that are an indication for active treatment are troublesome lymphadenopathy and significant liver or spleen enlargement.

Steroids can also be used if there is severe anaemia or a very low platelet count. For deposits in bone that cause symptoms referral to a radiotherapist is indicated for localized irradiation.

Acute leukaemias of the lymphatic, myeloid or monoblastic type are uncommon in the elderly. They are usually the sequel of chronic leukaemias and rarely occur *de novo*. Treatment is with cytotoxic therapy and demands referral to an oncologist. The results of treatment are very poor, and in the authors' opinion such treatment is very rarely indicated.

Aplastic anaemia, agranulocytosis and leucopaenia

Marrow depression producing *aplastic anaemia* may occasionally be seen in the elderly. Sometimes the cause is never found, but drug-induced aplasia must be excluded. Aplastic anaemia generally denotes a depression of all cell types in the bone marrow. The prognosis of the idiopathic type is very poor and it rarely responds to steroid treatment. Drug-induced aplasia often recovers after the offending drug is withdrawn, but until recovery has taken place it is wise to give steroids in high dosage, e.g. prednisolone 60 mg daily.

Agranulocytosis and leucopaenia are generally caused by drugs. The chief offenders are the antidepressants, tranquillizers and some antibiotics. Carbimazole and cytotoxic agents will also produce a similar picture. Infections may cause major problems in these patients and as far as possible exposure to infection should be avoided. Withdrawal of the drug will usually result in recovery.

SUMMARY

Anaemias are common in the elderly. Iron deficiency anaemia is most frequently seen and is usually due to blood loss. In addition to correcting the anaemia the cause must be found and treated appropriately. Nutritional anaemia is more likely to be of the vitamin B_{12} or folic acid deficiency type,

123

although iron deficiency and scurvy do still occur in westernized society. The appropriate blood levels need to be requested and treatment given with the relevant product. Less common causes of anaemia of these types are hypothyroidism and gastric and small bowel disease.

Of the leukaemias the chronic lymphatic type is the most common. This is generally benign and requires no treatment. Acute leukaemias are unusual and are often the end-stage of chronic leukaemia: treatment is generally not indicated. Myeloproliferative disease may be found and requires a bone marrow sample for its proper identification. Treatment is supportive with venesection and radioactive phosphorus for polycythaemia, and blood transfusions for myelofibrosis.

THYROID DISORDERS

Disease of the thyroid gland is important in the elderly and occurs in up to three per cent of this age group. Underactivity of the thyroid is about five times as common as overactivity with an equal distribution between the sexes. Thyroid disease of either type may be extremely difficult to recognize and is an example of the value of routine blood screening in the elderly.

Hypothyroidism (myxoedema)

This is the most important thyroid disorder in the elderly. It may be the result of an autoimmune thyroiditis (Hashimoto's), hypopituitarism or previous thyroid ablation either by surgery or, more commonly, radioactive iodine. Drug treatment of thyrotoxicosis with carbimazole may also cause hypothyroidism.

Myxoedema may present in a number of ways. Most patients become very lethargic, with slowing of both mental and physical functions. Constipation is usual and most patients gain weight. Memory is impaired and some patients may be extremely confused and psychotic (myxoedema madness). Intolerance of cold is marked and these patients wear an inappropriate amount of clothes. Erythema *ab igne* on the shins is often a coincidental sign in these patients. Hypothermia may occur. In severe and previously unrecognized cases myxoedema coma may be found. Occasionally myxoedema may present as a carpal tunnel syndrome due to trapping of the median nerve by the oedematous flexor retinaculum at the wrist.

The clinical features of advanced myxoedema are well known. They include the puffy face due to mucoid deposition in the skin. The outer third of the eyebrows may be lost and the hair is coarse and dry. The voice is hoarse because of the thickened vocal cords. The myocardium may be involved and leads to intractable heart failure, bradycardia and often conduction disturbances. The tendon reflexes, especially the ankle jerk, have a characteristically slow relaxation phase.

The diagnosis of myxoedema is made by measuring the thyroid function tests, the serum T_4 is reduced and the serum TSH is raised in the absence of hypopituitarism. The thyroid auto-antibodies will be raised in Hashimoto's disease. The ECG may show a sinus bradycardia, conduction disturbances and in severe cases there will be generalized T wave inversion. The QRS comlexes are generally of low voltage.

Management

Once the diagnosis of myxoedema is established replacement treatment with thyroxine should be started. Initially it is usually reasonable to commence with a dose of 50 μg daily, but in very old frail patients, especially if there is evidence of myocardial involvement, the initial dose can be reduced to 25 μg daily. After two to three weeks the dose of thyroid replacement can be doubled and thereafter increased by 50 μg increments until adequate replacement is given. The usual replacement dose is between 100 and 200 μg daily.

The hormone replacement should only be given once a day. The measurement of adequate hormone replacement is assessed by repeatedly measuring the serum TSH level: there is no point in measuring the serum T_4 level in patients on replacement therapy. Follow-up should be for life and it is the responsibility of the consultant or general practitioner to operate an effective recall system for these patients.

Patients who have heart failure due to myxoedematous myocardial disease are extremely difficult to treat and often respond poorly to hormone replacement and anti-failure therapy. Bed rest is essential in these cases and it may be preferable to admit the patient to hospital.

Hyperthyroidism

Overactivity of the thyroid is usually a result of uni- or multi-nodular goitre. Graves' disease is not common in the elderly. Thus the symptoms of hyperthyroidism in the elderly may be more difficult to identify than in the young.

Weight loss and heat intolerance are almost universal. Atrial fibrillation, either established or paroxysmal, is usually present in the elderly hyperthyroid patient. The eye signs of Graves' disease are often absent, and thus proptosis and lid lag are rarely seen. Tremor of the outstretched hands and agitation are also often absent. Many patients complain of palpitations or a rapid heart action. The term 'masked hyperthyroidism' has been coined to describe this situation in the elderly, when the only abnormal signs are weight loss and atrial fibrillation. 'Apathetic hyperthyroidism' may also occur, when agitation and restlessness are absent and the patient is withdrawn.

The diagnosis is confirmed by finding elevation of the serum T_4 level. If there is any doubt about the diagnosis a TRH stimulation test should be performed, where it is found that the level of serum TSH is not significantly raised by intravenous injection of TRH.

Management

Once the diagnosis is confirmed the patient should be immediately referred to a radiotherapist for treatment with radioactive iodine. This is a fairly rapid and permanent treatment and is ideal for the older patient in whom there is no significant risk of leukaemia developing as a late result of the radioactive drug. In the meantime it is usually necessary to start treatment with a beta-blocking agent, such as propranolol (Inderal) 10 mg tds. This treatment will control the tremor and restlessness and help to lower the heart rate. The dose of beta-blocker may need to be increased until these symptoms are controlled in some cases. If established atrial fibrillation is present it is usually associated with a high ventricular rate; in these cases digoxin should be given, with a starting dose of 0.25 mg twice daily for two days and then 0.125 mg daily. If the atrial fibrillation is paroxysmal it is better to give an anti-arrhythmic agent, such as amiodarone (Cordarone) in a starting dose of 200 mg tds for two weeks, then reducing to 400 mg daily for a further two weeks and after that a maintenance dose of 200 mg daily. Amiodarone is a very effective drug in the control of paroxysmal atrial arrhythmias, but is associated with several side-effects that require careful monitoring. It usually has a depressing effect on thyroid function, since it is an iodinated compound and blocks the uptake of T_4. This effect, however, does not remove the need to give proper doses of radioactive iodine, although the iodine should only be given after three days of no amiodarone treatment. Amiodarone also may interfere with liver function and can cause parkinsonian-like tremor and rigidity, although these effects are related to high blood levels. Some patients may get photosensitivity rashes if exposed to the sun. Despite this formidable list of possible complications, at the time of writing amiodarone is the most effective agent for preventing paroxysms of atrial fibrillation.

Treatment of hyperthyroidism by surgery, or drugs such as carbimazole, in elderly patients is very rarely indicated.

Patients who have received radioactive iodine treatment are usually controlled within four to six weeks. Unfortunately the long-term incidence of secondary myxoedema is very high and all these patients should be monitored for the rest of their life by means of T_4 and TSH measurements in the serum. If they are found to be myxoedematous replacement thyroid should be given as described for myxoedema above.

Non-toxic goitres

Non-toxic goitres may be seen in any age group and are produced by oversecretion of TSH. Sometimes they may be very large. By definition the output of thyroid hormone is normal. The most important cause is lack of iodine in the diet. Non-toxic goitre can also occur in auto-immune thyroiditis. These goitres may be induced by several drugs, including para-amino salicylic acid, phenylbutazone, iodine-containing expectorant mixtures, tolbutamide, carbimazole and thiouracil.

Management

The offending cause should be identified and corrected, whether by increasing the iodine in the diet or stopping the relevant drug.

Carcinomas of the thyroid

These are uncommon diseases in the elderly. The majority are papillary carcinomas: less often seen are the follicular carcinomas. Their natural history is extremely variable, from being benign to very malignant. They may spread locally or metastasise to the bones, lungs or brain. They are most often a cause of a solitary thyroid nodule, and on finding such a nodule, it is important to refer the patient for a thyroid scan.

Treatment of thyroid carcinoma is by total thyroidectomy followed by radioactive iodine ablation. Following this procedure replacement thyroid hormone will have to be given. This treatment also helps to suppress TSH production and is important since some of these tumours are hormone-dependent.

DIABETES MELLITUS

Diabetes mellitus should be regarded as a description rather than a diagnosis. It describes a state of chronic hyperglycaemia and is usually associated with other clinical and biochemical abnormalities. Hyperglycaemia indicates fasting blood sugar levels of greater than 8 mmol/l or postabsorptive blood glucose in excess of 11 mmol/l.

Aetiology

Diabetes exists in at least 2% of the elderly population. The majority of elderly patients have Type II or non-insulin dependent diabetes. A very much smaller proportion of elderly people have Type I or insulin-dependent diabetes, whether those who have survived with this condition into old age or the very few people who develop this condition in old age.

The major factor in the development of non insulin-dependent diabetes is obesity. These patients may have a high circulating insulin level and both receptor and post-receptor abnormalities. No single nutritional component is especially diabetogenic, although iron overload in some Africans may lead to pancreatic fibrosis, and spoiled cassava consumption in chronically malnourished people may be found in India which also leads to pancreatic fibrosis. There is increased genetic predisposition, but no recognized mode of inheritance or HLA association.

Type I diabetes is much more likely to have a genetic susceptibility, and almost 50% of diabetic sibling pairs are HLA identical.

Clinical features

The clinical presentation of diabetes will depend on the type. The development of significant weight loss with polyuria and polydipsia, ketosis and pre-coma or coma are all features of Type I diabetes and are unusually seen for the first time in elderly patients. The majority of elderly patients will present with rather innocuous symptoms, such as malaise, slight weight loss and, often, polyuria and polydipsia of mild degree. In most cases the diagnosis is made either on routine urinalysis or on random blood sugar screening. Glycosuria may not necessarily be present.

The complications of diabetes are often found in Type II diabetes and may well be the presenting feature of the disease in the elderly. These complications may be complex and produce symptoms that are frequently seen in old people. They may be classified as follows:

Complication	Symptoms/Signs
Retinopathy	
Mild background retinopathy	none
Background retinopathy with macular oedema	loss of visual acuity
Proliferative retinopathy	none
	loss of visual acuity
	sudden blindness (vitreous haemorrhage)
Advanced diabetic eye disease	loss of visual acuity
	blindness
Neuropathy	
Symmetrical polyneuropathy:	
Sensory polyneuropathy	none
	pain and paraesthesiae (especially feet)
Autonomic neuropathy	postural hypotension
	neurogenic bladder
	diarrhoea
	impotence
	bradycardia
	gustatory sweating
	gastroparesis
Mononeuropathy and multiple mononeuropathy	loss of eye movement (especially cranial nerves III & VI)
	carpal tunnel
(Radiculopathy, cranial nerve lesions, isolated peripheral nerve lesions)	foot drop
	painful limbs
	painless trauma
Diabetic amyotrophy	severe pain
	muscle wasting
Arterial disease	
Major vessel ischaemia	strokes
	angina/myocardial infarction
	leg gangrene
Small vesel disease	renal disease (proteinuria, renal failure)
	diabetic foot (ulcers and gangrene of toes)

Diabetic retinopathy is an important cause of blindness in the UK and accounts for over 14% of all blind registrations. These complications are seen in most Type I diabetics after they have had the disease for 15 years or more, but may occur much earlier in Type II diabetes.

Mild background retinopathy may produce no symptoms in its early stages. The lesions consist of microaneurysms, hard exudates and cotton wool spots around the macular area. These lesions progress with time and all suspected and known diabetics should have regular and careful fundoscopic examination.

Maculopathy with background retinopathy is most often seen in the elderly non-insulin-dependent diabetics. Hard exudate rings or plaques develop lateral to the macula and advance towards it causing progressive loss of vision. The elderly often do not volunteer the symptoms of visual loss and examination of visual acuity should be regularly made in these patients. The situation is further complicated by the fact that there may be maculopathy with little to see on ophthalmoscopy. In these cases fluoroscein angiography is indicated.

Proliferative retinopathy is more likely to occur in younger insulin-dependent diabetics, but may also be seen in the elderly. In this condition there is aggressive new vessel formation. Symptoms may be absent initially, but if vitreous haemorrhage occurs there may be sudden loss of vision.

Advanced diabetic eye disease is the end-stage of retinopathy. This may be due to vitreous haemorrhage, advanced fibrous tissue formation, as part of the new vessel formation, or thrombotic glaucoma. This latter condition is caused by new vessel formation on the iris and leads to outflow obstruction from the anterior chamber and raised intra-ocular pressure. It produces painful visual field loss and ultimately blindness.

Diabetic neuropathy occurs in about 15% of elderly diabetics. Pressure palsies are more common in diabetics and can produce compression of the median nerve at the wrist (carpal tunnel syndrome), isolated foot drop and cranial nerve palsies, usually of the III and VI nerves causing disturbance of ocular movements.

Sensory neuropathy may be multiple and is often symmetrical. In the early stages there may be no symptoms, but pain and paraesthesiae are common and usually occur in a glove and stocking distribution, although the feet are more commonly affected than the hands. Loss of light touch sensation may cause difficulty in handling small objects such as needles and buttons, and the problem is compounded if there is loss of visual acuity due to retinopathy. Sensory neuropathy may be limited to the loss of the ankle jerk. In more advanced cases painless trauma may cause problems with the feet and this is also compounded if there is associated diabetic peripheral vascular damage. More rarely neuropathic joints (Charcot) may occur, especially the ankle joint. Motor neuropathy is most unusual in diabetics and muscular weakness and wasting are rarely seen.

Autonomic neuropathy is a common problem in the elderly and diabetes is a major cause. It may often be associated with peripheral neuropathy. The most frequently found problem in autonomic neuropathy is postural hypotension. The bladder may also be affected and this is an important cause of incontinence. Less frequently cardiac and respiratory denervation may occur and give rise to bradycardia and respiratory arrests during or after anaesthesia.

The vascular complications of diabetes may affect the major arteries of the heart and brain, but the major problems caused by diabetes in the elderly affect the smaller vesels. The kidneys may be involved and proteinuria may be the first abnormal finding. Progressively impaired renal function occurs which may alter the threshold for glucose excretion and further complicate the control of the elderly diabetic. Ultimately renal failure occurs. If there is associated hypertension, this must be carefully controlled.

The diabetic foot is the most frequently seen complication in the elderly diabetic and is due to a combination of vascular and neuropathic disease. Chronic painless ulcers occur, especially over pressure areas. These ulcers usually become infected and may lead to deep abscess formation and osteomyelitis, especially of the head of the first metatarsal bone. Painful ischaemic changes may also occur in the foot and may only involve one or more toes. These may become gangrenous even though the foot pulses are normal. Other problems that may occur in the diabetic foot include painless burns from fires and hot water bottles, friction ulcers from ill-fitting shoes and infection from careless chiropody. Major deformity of the foot may occur due to bony disintegration or joint dislocation and exacerbate further ulceration or pressure damage to the foot.

Management

Establishing the diagnosis

It is essential to establish the diagnosis of the diabetic state firmly. This can be done usually by measuring the fasting glucose level, which should normally be below 8 mmol/1, and by measuring the glucose level two hours after a full meal or a 75 mg oral glucose load when the level should be below 11 mmol/l. It is rarely necessary to go to the trouble of exposing the patient to a full oral glucose tolerance test unless the blood glucose levels mentioned above are equivocal.

Blood sugar control

Since the majority of elderly diabetics have Type II disease every effort should be made to control the weight by dietary restriction as well as to limit the glucose intake. This is usually much more easily said than done, and careful counselling of both patient and relatives is essential. The considerable time that needs to be spent on these matters will repay itself amply by better control and the minimalization of later complications.

It is unrealistic to suppose that elderly patients can easily change a lifetime's dietary habit. A suitable diet will have to be constructed for each individual patient based as far as possible on the individual's food pattern. The spacing of meals is important and slowly absorbed unrefined high-fibre carbohydrates, such as bread, potatoes, pasta and fruit, should form the basis of normal carbohydrate intake. Rapidly absorbed sugars should be avoided and reserved for hypoglycaemic states only. Dietary fat should be restricted, especially saturated fatty foods. This may be more difficult if there is unreasonable restriction of carbohydrate in the diet. Obsessive aims at continual normoglycaemia in the elderly can produce unnecessary misery, and are probably inappropriate unless there are major diabetic complications.

The majority of elderly diabetics will be adequately controlled by these simple dietary measures and associated weight reduction. Assessment of control is best done by regular sampling of venous blood, as in many old people the renal threshold for glucose is disturbed and glucose in the urine may only appear with very high blood glucose levels. It is a good routine to get diabetics regularly to test their urine, whatever their renal threshold for glucose, as this helps to reinforce the overall control of their diabetic state. For those patients who have difficulty in manipulating testing of urine, dipstick testing (e.g. Diastix) is preferable. If there are visual complications it will be necessary for a relative or nurse to do the testing. A few patients will be able to test their own capillary blood samples at home using one of the portable devices currently available, which rely on the development of colour following the timed application of blood on to an enzyme-tipped strip.

If the elderly diabetic is not controlled by dietary measures the next step is to introduce oral treatment for Type II diabetes.

Oral hypoglycaemic agents

Sulphonylureas

Tolbutamide	Short acting, mild action
Chlorpropamide	Long acting (24 hours+), potent, antidiuretic
Glibenclamide	Medium acting, potent, diuretic
Gliquidone	Sulphonylurea of choice in renal failure
Others (e.g. glipizide, glibornuride, glymidine, etc.)	Similar to glibenclamide

Biguanides

Metformin
Phenformin
} Risk of lactic acidosis

The sulphonylureas act primarily by stimulating insulin release, but also have some hepatic and peripheral hypoglycaemic action. They are all potentiated by, and in some cases, potentiate, the concurrent administration of sulphonamides, beta-blocking drugs, anticoagulants and monoamine-oxidase inhibitors. Tolbutamide (Rastinon) 500 mg–1 g bd or tds is the safest drug for the elderly because of its mild action and rare induction of hypoglycaemic attacks. If this drug fails to produce adequate control chlorpropamide (Diabenese) 100–250 mg daily or glibenclamide (Daonil) 5–20 mg daily may be used. Both these drugs may be potent enough to cause hypoglycaemia and the patient should be warned of this complication and the symptoms carefully explained to him.

The biguanide group of agents act in several ways to produce hypoglycaemia by interfering with absorption, hepatic metabolism and peripheral potentiation of the effects of insulin. They may cause lactic acidosis especially in the presence of renal and hepatic disease and with alcohol ingestion.

Phenformin is now contra-indicated and is no longer available in Britain. The risk of lactic acidosis is considerably less with metformin, but this drug should not be used in patients with significant renal or hepatic impairment. Metformin (Glucophage) may be sufficient on its own to control an obese diabetic or it can be used in combination with a sulphonylurea in a dose of 500–1700 mg daily.

Insulin

The majority of elderly patients do not require insulin treatment. The indications for insulin treatment include the newly diagnosed diabetic with major complications or infections or those with no obesity, significant thirst and polyuria and ketosis. The recognition of such situations is often an indication to admit the patient to hospital for initial control and treatment of the complications. This may be avoided if there is a diabetic liaison nurse from the hospital diabetic clinic. To ensure adequate and rapid control short-acting insulins should be used, usually by infusion pump. These techniques are for hospital staff and will not be further discussed.

Once the patient has been controlled in hospital and has been discharged, home continued insulin may in some cases be necessary. If the insulin requirements of an elderly patient are below 40 units daily it is probably preferable to use a long-acting single dose insulin either singly (e.g. isophane) or in combination (e.g. semilente and ultralente). If the insulin requirements are greater than 40 units daily or the patient is poorly controlled on single injections, it is wise to use twice daily injections of shorter acting insulins, or possibly combined short and intermediate mixtures of insulin.

Older patients may have considerable difficulty in managing their own injections and if relatives cannot be taught to help, or are unavailable, it will be necessary to get the district nurses to manage their injections. Patients can be helped by providing plastic syringes with integral needles on them and by providing filling stops on the syringes if they have difficulty in loading the insulin because of visual or arthritic problems.

Management of complications

With all the complications of diabetes it is essential to ensure the best possible control of the blood sugar. This may involve changing the patient either from oral agents to insulin for this period or increasing the frequency of insulin injections using shorter acting preparations. It may be impossible to achieve these aims in the home situation and in these circumstances it will be necessary to admit the patient to hospital for a time. The situation is most likely to obtain when the patient develops an acute infection or gangrenous changes in the feet. The introduction of the diabetic liaison nurse in some hospital diabetic clinics may reduce the need for hospital admission.

Eye complications

The development of xenon arc and, more recently, argon laser photocoagulation has revolutionized the management of diabetic maculopathy and proliferative retinopathy. It is important to refer the patient to an ophthalmologist early before the vision has deteriorated to 6/24. Once the vision has deteriorated beyond 6/36 the results of treatment are pretty unsatisfactory. Thus regular assessment of both fundoscopic changes and visual acuity are essential. The development of vitreous haemorrhage, fibrous tissue and glaucoma are urgent indications for referral to an eye surgeon.

Neuropathy

Unfortunately the prognosis of diabetic neuropathy does not appear to be improved even by perfect diabetic control. In these situations careful attention must be given to explaining the dangers of pressure damage to the feet, and nail and callus care, to the patient and his attendants. General foot care is an important part of the work of district nurses and health visitors. The treatment of ulceration and sepsis requires skilled nursing attention and if necessary systemic antibiotics after swabs have been taken for culture to the laboratory. Any foot sepsis that does not quickly settle with treatment should alert the doctor to the development of abscess formation and osteomyelitis. Radiography may help to elucidate this situation and the patient should be referred to the orthopaedic surgeon. Ischaemic changes in the toes may not cause pain and can be safely observed and managed at home. If pain is a problem the patient should be referred to a surgeon. Peripheral vasodilators and vascular surgical reconstruction are rarely helpful in these conditions and are not indicated. Infection and gangrenous changes in the feet or elsewhere are likely to upset the blood sugar control and will require monitoring and, if necessary, alteration in treatment.

Autonomic neuropathy giving rise to postural hypotension cannot be reversed but the patient can be considerably helped by simple measures, such as supplying elastic supportive stockings and general advice about rising slowly from sitting or lying positions.

The management of neurogenic bladder is discussed on pp. 100-1.

SUMMARY

Diabetes is a common problem in the elderly. It is usually associated with obesity and responds well to weight and dietary control. Oral hypoglycaemic and, sometimes, insulin preparations may be necessary for the adequate control that will minimize the symptoms and long-term complications that occur in diabetics. The management of diabetes is an excellent example of how effective the proper use of the primary health care team can be, and in most cases patients should not need to be referred to hospital. The development of infections and complications involving the eye or peripheral vascular system requires careful monitoring and, often, referral to a hospital specialist. In all aspects of the disease there should be very full co-operation between the patient, relatives, nurse and doctor to ensure optimum management.

Each practice should have a system for identifying and monitoring the diabetic patients on its list. Only in this way can the condition be effectively controlled and the risk of complications minimized. Systems based on loose-leaf books, card indices and microcomputers have all been shown to fulfil this function satisfactorily.

PSYCHIATRIC DISORDERS

Psychiatric disturbances in the elderly are extremely common and will present the general practitioner with some of his most difficult problems.

The incidence of psychiatric disorders in the population at home over the age of 65 years is around 5%. However, by the age of 80 years the incidence of significant mental illness rises to over 20%. This situation is brought about by two main factors. There is progressive neuronal loss with rising age which results in progressive brain failure. In addition, the effects of ageing in other body systems lead to a deterioration in the ability to maintain an independent existence and reduce the individual's tolerance of stress and disease. These effects are heightened by the general loss of status in the elderly in western society, insecurity and loss of interest after retirement, fears of death and disability and death of friends and relatives.

Dementia

Dementia, or chronic brain failure, is characterised by significant loss of neurones and brain substance leading to an irreversible global loss of intellectual function.

Dementia is the single most important mental illness in old age and occurs in 10% of all people over 65 years and by the age of 80 years the incidence rises to about 20%.

There are various types of dementia:

Presenile
Senile

Arteriosclerotic (multi-infarct)
Mixed senile and arteriosclerotic
Secondary (myxoedema, vitamin B_{12} deficiency, folate deficiency, etc)

From a management point of view the only advantage of differentiating the type of the dementia is to be able to give some accurate estimation of prognosis since, by definition, the disease is irreversible. The only exception to this rule is in the case of secondary dementia, where it is sometimes possible to produce some improvement by treating the primary cause if it is found early enough.

Presenile dementia is associated with Alzheimer's and Pick's disease and Huntington's chorea. By definition these dementias start to manifest themselves before the age of 65 years, but may first present to the general practitioner after that age. These diseases are rare and rapidly progressive once significant brain failure is recognised.

Senile (primary neuronal) dementia accounts for about one half of all cases. In this condition there is a substantial loss of neurones and thinning of the cerebral cortex with widening of the sulci and shrinkage of the gyri. It is not known whether this is an exaggerated form of the normal ageing process or a separate disease entity. Electron microscopy of the brain shows a proliferation of senile plaques and neurofibrillary tangles. Biochemical tests demonstrate a loss of neurotransmitters and some enzyme changes.

Multi-infarct or arteriosclerotic dementia is often associated with previous hypertension and widespread arteriosclerosis.

Secondary dementias are probably not true dementias since they are, to some extent, reversible when the primary disease is controlled. The most important causes of secondary dementia are hypovitaminosis of B_{12}, folic acid deficiency and myxoedema. Depletion of many B vitamins, especially thiamine, may occur in alcoholics and produce a similar picture which is to some extent reversible on withdrawal of the alcohol and repletion with massive doses of B vitamins.

Clinical features

The cardinal clinical features are the same for all the dementias:

Memory loss
Confusion and disorders of behaviour
Intellectual impairment
Personality disintegration

Memory loss principally affects recent memory, whilst distant memory is well preserved until the late stages of the disease. This represents a marked exaggeration of the normal recent memory loss of ageing.

Confusion and disorders of behaviour are generally secondary to the memory loss. The confusion manifests itself in a number of ways; there is disorientation in time and, often, in space. Mealtimes may be forgotten and in patients living alone this may lead to secondary neglect and weight loss. Belongings are often mislaid and clothes are put on in a haphazard and inappropriate fashion. This confusion may lead to severe anxiety and frustration. Sometimes patients become very aggressive or, conversely, withdrawn. Paranoid features are common and people will be accused of stealing belongings that have been mislaid. In the later stages of the disease socially unacceptable behaviour occurs and patients may urinate and defaecate in inappropriate places. Wandering is common, and if this is associated with sexual exposure, may cause a public nuisance.

Intellectual impairment is progressive. The main problem is the failure to grasp new ideas and to learn. This is especially a problem if the patient develops a mobility problem since they are unable to cope with the learning techniques that are part of the rehabilitation programme. The combination of intellectual impairment and confusion and memory loss makes normal conversation with friends and relatives increasingly difficult and ultimately leads to increasing social isolation. This in turn accelerates the development of behaviour problems.

Progressive disintegration of the personality is characteristic of dementia. Personality traits that have been present in earlier life become exaggerated and it is usually the worst features of these that emerge more strongly. Gradually the patient becomes divorced from reality and fails to recognize that there is a problem.

If the patient is living with someone else the early features of dementia can be absorbed and coped with. Often close relatives may not recognize the scale of the problem. However, as time passes the dement becomes more and more difficult to live with and the frustration and demands on the carer become overwhelming and may induce mental or physical problems in them. If a demented patient lives alone the breakdown of the home situation occurs earlier. Self neglect, disorganization within the home and wandering may become very severe before the situation is appreciated by others. The police may become involved by accusations of stealing or when there is wandering in the streets: in these circumstances the situation can very rapidly get badly out of control and may force admission to an institution under an order.

Management

The management of the demented patient may prove extremely difficult and time-consuming. The first task for the doctor is to make sure that the diagnosis is correct. This will involve taking a history not only from the patient but also from friends and relatives. A careful physical examination should be made and blood screening should include full blood count, electrolytes, blood glucose, serum B_{12} and folate, calcium and syphilis serology. Thyroid function tests are essential. It is also wise to make some formal assessment of mental function in order to establish a baseline for monitoring progress. A simple test of mental function is Hodkinson's modification of the RCP test.

Abbreviated RCP test

(1) Age
(2) Time (to the nearest hour)
(3) Address (for recall at the end of the test)
  e.g. 42 West Street, Crawley
(4) Year
(5) Name of local hospital
(6) Recognition of two persons by role, not name (doctor, nurse, etc)
(7) Date of birth
(8) Year of First World War (either 1914 or 1918)
(9) Name of present monarch or president
(10) Count backwards from 20 to 1. Then recall (3).

Depression may sometimes be confused with dementia. Not infrequently they coexist together. Apathy, neglect, memory loss and incontinence occur in both conditions. Depression tends to be of more acute onset and the memory loss is patchy. Since the two are sometimes difficult to differentiate it is often worthwhile giving these patients a trial of antidepressant drugs.

Toxic confusional states may sometimes be mistaken for dementia. In toxic states, however, the onset is usually acute and in addition to the confusion there may be clouding of consciousness. Hallucinations may be severe, and are not usually seen in dementia. There is usually fever and other signs of infection. Biochemical testing will also exclude or confirm the presence of hypo- or hyper-glycaemia, uraemia and hypercalcaemia. It is important to recognise these toxic states since prompt treatment will ensure a rapid return to mental normality.

Psychotic states such as paraphrenia may have some of the features of dementia, but memory is not impaired and the intellect is well preserved.

When the diagnosis of dementia is established it is vital to discuss the situation and the likely prognosis with the relatives. It is best if it is possible to keep the patient in their own home, since moving to a new environment will make the confusion worse. Relatives and friends will need continued support and counselling if they are to cope with the demanding life that they will have to undergo in order to keep the patient reasonably well at home. Regular visits from the doctor will be appreciated. Visits and assistance with the physical needs from the district nurse are essential. Home helps and meals on wheels services will be of great benefit if the patient is alone for much of the time.

The availability of day care and visits to luncheon clubs will be of great benefit in the earlier stages of the disease. In later stages, however, the removal of the patient to a strange environment may accentuate the confusion. Sometimes 'holiday beds' in a residential home or hospital may afford much needed relief to the carers, and these should be generally available through the local social services department of the hospital.

There is little evidence that *drug treatment* has any effect on the course of the disease. However, since the prognosis is so gloomy it is often worth trying a course of such drugs as naftidrofuryl (Praxilene) 200 mg tds, dihydroergot alkaloids (Hydergine) 4.5 mg daily or isoxsuprine (Duvadilan) 40 mg bd. Occasionally a worthwhile improvement may occur.

Behaviour and sleep disturbances can be helped considerably by giving short-acting hypnotics, such as temazepam (Normison) 10–20 mg or chlormethiazole (Heminevrin) 0.5–1.0 g at night. If there are significant behaviour disturbances at night despite these drugs it is worth adding a tranquillizer such as thioridazine (Melleril) 25–75 mg or promazine (Sparine) 50–100 mg. The long-acting hypnotics such as nitrazepam are contra-indicated in the elderly, although they are extremely popular: they cause a hangover effect and make the patient drowsy and often confused the following morning.

Daytime behaviour problems and agitation should be treated with drugs such as thioridazine (Melleril) 10–50 mg tds. In severe cases the use of haloperidol (Serenace) 0.5–1.5 mg tds or chlorpromazine (Largactil) 25–50 mg tds may be helpful, although they are likely to cause significant drowsiness and parkinsonian symptoms. The latter side effects can be controlled with the concomitant administration of orphenadrine (Disipal) 25 mg tds. The benzodiazepine group of drugs, such as diazepam, are best not used for demented patients during the day. Alcohol should be avoided.

Thus the management of the demented patient will be principally supportive. The family doctor plays an important co-ordinating role in this condition and will need to enlist the help of many people including psychiatrists, nurses, social workers and statutory and voluntary home care workers. The aim should be to keep the patient in his own environment if at all possible. Sometimes there is confusion about which hospital specialist to call in to help these patients. Many hospital specialists try to avoid getting involved in these situations and there is often a 'buck-passing' attitude taken by consultants and their junior staff. A reasonable guide, that has been accepted by the Royal College of Psychiatrists and the British Geriatrics Society, is that if the demented patient is ambulant he should be within the province of a psychiatrist, but if he is demented and non-ambulant then he is the responsibility of the physician in geriatric medicine.

Depression

Depression is a common and important disorder of the elderly. It occurs in as many as 15% of those over 65 years. Successful suicide is much more common in late life than in younger patients and, therefore, the illness should be recognized early and treated vigorously.

The clinical features of depression in the elderly are similar to those in the young. Apathy and lack of energy are almost universal and the sleep is also disturbed. Difficulty in getting off to sleep suggests reactive depression and early morning waking suggests the endogenous variety. The appetite is poor and these patients lose weight and are constipated. Sometimes they are incontinent of urine and often exhibit signs of self-neglect. Sadness and tearfulness are obvious signs, but sudden mood swings and inappropriate laughing and crying are more likely to be due to cerebrovascular disease and are not features of depression. Depressed patients may have some recent memory loss but are not hallucinated or deluded or confused. Sometimes depressed patients have associated agitation and anxiety. The disease may also occur in combination with dementia.

Management

Psychotherapy will help many old people. Depression is often precipitated by social isolation, bereavement, retirement, removal from their own home and loss of status. These patients need time, encouragement and sympathy. Busy family doctors may find that they just do not have the time to spend with the patient that they should. In these situations it is essential to enlist the help of others, including health visitors and psychiatric social workers and nurses. Visits to day centres and luncheon clubs may be of help to a number of patients.

If no improvement is rapidly made with the above simple measures resort must be taken to antidepressant drugs. Each doctor has his favourite drug, but in the opinion of the authors the tricyclic agents are the most effective in the elderly. Imipramine (Tofranil) 10 mg tds and 25–50 mg at night is often very effective but no significant improvement can be expected for two to three weeks at least. Protryptiline (Concordin) in an initial dose of 5 mg tds may have a more rapid onset of action. For those who show marked emotional lability clomipramine (Anafranil) 5–10 mg tds is very effective. Amitriptyline (Tryptizol) 10–25 mg tds and 50 mg at night is a very effective agent and has the advantage of having some tranquillizing action for those who have anxiety as well.

For those patients who are severely depressed and who do not respond to antidepressant drugs one should consider ECT treatment and help must be sought from the psychiatrist. There is no major contra-indications to ECT and age alone is no barrier to giving this form of treatment.

Alcoholism

Alcoholism is much more common in the elderly than is generally realized. It has been estimated that the incidence is as high as 9% of those over 65 years. Many of these patients are women. About one half of these patients have been heavy drinkers in younger life. In the rest drinking starts late in life, often as a response to bereavement, social isolation or other social disaster. Some of these patients have significant depression. Many are extremely devious about their drinking habits and their means of obtaining alcohol. Few patients will admit to excessive drinking.

The management of alcoholism does not differ in the old from that practised in the young. It is essential to withdraw alcohol completely as brain damage is seriously threatened. The withdrawal must be covered with oral chlormethiazole (Heminevrin) 0.5 g four times daily initially and reducing over 10 to 14 days. It is also wise to give full doses of multivitamins of the B complex, preferably by intravenous injections of Parentrovite daily.

In serious cases, or where the home circumstances are unsatisfactory, it is probably better to admit the patient to a psychiatric unit initially.

After the initial 'drying out' phase long-term support and counselling is necessary. Many patients will benefit by joining Alcoholics Anonymous.

The Diogenes syndrome

The Diogenes syndrome is a bizarre condition which most family doctors will encounter in their practice. The syndrome is characterized by virtual withdrawal from society, living in extreme squalor, rejecting all forms of

142

medical and social assistance and the collecting and hoarding of rubbish (syllogomania). It occurs equally in men and women and usually in those of previously high social standing. Most of the patients are intelligent and often reasonably well off financially. Professional people seem to be extremely susceptible to this condition. It may be precipitated by either retirement or bereavement. These patients do not have any significant psychiatric disturbance and are not alcoholic. There is often a history of eccentricity. Many of these people are not known to the medical and social services departments and, indeed, usually turn these helping people away if they call. The home is usually recognizable from the outside by the appearance of squalor and neglect, with unkempt gardens, broken windows and dirty and torn curtains in an otherwise smart area. Entry to the home may be impeded by mountains of rubbish, newspapers and rotting food.

The majority of these patients present for the first time as an acute medical emergency requiring admission to hospital. In addition to an acute chest infection or stroke, there are usually signs of chronic malnutrition and anaemia. The mortality rate for women is especially high and in the region of 60%. Sometimes the patient may be seen by the doctor and refuse admission to hospital and it may be necessary to force admission under a court order, especially if there is a danger to the health and safety of other people. After the acute illness forcing the admission to hospital has been treated and the patient has been returned to his home, there is a very high relapse rate to the former condition. The doctor must try and persuade the patient to accept home help and support, but very often it will be vigorously refused.

Sleep disturbances

Most elderly patients will find sleeping a problem as they get older. It is especially likely to be a feature of psychiatric illnesses, such as depression and anxiety states. It is normal for the elderly to develop more fragmented sleep. It takes longer to get off to sleep and the 'slow wave' sleep is reduced with the result that waking periods in the night are both more frequent and longer than is found in younger people. Many patients compensate for this by taking longer and longer catnaps during the day. This may lead to a complete reversal of the normal diurnal sleep pattern.

The expectation of sleep may also present a problem for the elderly. After a lifetime of going to sleep with relative ease the elderly patient may have difficulty in adjusting to sleep problems that are a normal feature of old age. Four to six hours sleep a night should be sufficient for the elderly.

Management

At the first consultation about sleeping difficulties it is important to explain the normal features of sleep patterns with ageing. This may well alleviate the problem and will avoid the need for giving hypnotic drugs to many patients. Sleep disturbance may be the first sign of a significant anxiety or depressive state and careful questioning about other body functions and mood is important to exclude these.

If these simple measures do not cure the problem, it will be necessary to use hypnotic drugs. Of the many that are available only the short-acting drugs should be used. These include dichloralphenazone (Welldorm) 650–1300 mg, temazepam (Normison, Euhypnos) 10–20 mg and chlormethiazole (Heminevrin) 500–1000 mg at night. The longer acting drugs such as nitrazepam and diazepam should never be used in the elderly for sleep problems. The barbiturates should never be used. Short courses should be given initially before commiting the patient to long-term treatment with these agents.

For patients who have depression a nocturnal dose of an anti-depressant agent can be used, such as amitriptyline (Tryptizol) 50–75 mg. Sometimes a short-acting hypnotic drug may need to be given as well.

For those patients with dementia and sleeping problems where there may be severe nocturnal confusion and wandering, a short-acting hypnotic combined with a tranquillizing drug of the phenothiazine group, such as promazine (Sparine) 50–100 mg may be very useful. This should ensure rest both for the patient and his immediate relatives and neighbours.

Summary

Psychiatric disorders are a very common problem in the elderly. Dementias will cause the most problems for both doctors and relatives alike. Other causes of confusion states must be excluded and treated as far as possible. The management of dementia hinges upon supportive treatment for the family. The role of drug treatment is only useful for the behavioural problems that may be associated with the dementia.

Depression and anxiety are frequently seen in the elderly. Awareness of these diseases, especially if there has been recent bereavement, should result in very effective control of the symptoms. Psychotherapy and drug treatment may be time-consuming for the primary health care team, but the results will be very rewarding.

Alcoholism may be a feature of a reactive depressive illness or an exaggeration of former lifelong drinking habits. Some of these patients will require the additional help of specialized psychiatric departments and long-term support from psychiatric social workers and bodies such as Alcoholics Anonymous.

Index

aches and pains 22-3
ageing changes 5-7
agranulocytosis 123
alcoholism 142
allopurinol (Zyloric) 83
alphacalcidol (One-Alpha) 67-8
alprenolol 47
Alzheimer's disease 28, 137
ambulatory dynamic electrocardiography 50-2
amiloride (Midamor) 40, 46
aminophylline 58
amiodarone (Cordarone X) 52-3, 53, 54, 126
amitryptiline (Tryptizol) 112, 142, 144
amputation-stump pain 111
anabolic steroids 65
anaemia 114-24
   aetiology 114-15
   aplastic 123
   investigations 115-16, 119
   iron deficiency 116-17, 119
   macrocytic 117-19
   megaloblastic 117-19
   pernicious 117-18, 119
   normocytic/normochromic 119
aneurysm 44, 45
angina, management 47-8
angiotensin-converting enzyme inhibitors 41, 60
ankle oedema 19-20
anxiety state 28
apathy 28-9
arthritis, septic 76
aspirin 47, 77
   + dipyridamole (Persantin) 47, 90

atenolol (Tenormin) 40, 48
atrial fibrillation 52-3
atrial premature complexes 53
atrioventricular block 54
autonomic instability 22

back pain 112-13
Baker's cyst 76, 81
barbiturates 144
bendrofluazide (Neo-NaClex) 40
bendrofluazide + potassium (Neo-NaClex-K) 59
benzhexol (Artane) 95
beta-blocking agents 9, 40, 47, 126
bethanidine 41
bladder problems 100-2
blood pressure, rise with age 35
bone disease 4, 61
bone tumours 71-4
Bornholm disease (Coxsackie B myalgia) 45
breathlessness 16-18
bromocriptine (Parlodel) 95-6
bumetanide (Burinex) 40, 46, 58, 59
bundle branch block 54
busulphan (Myleran) 122
bypass coronary surgery 48

calcitonin 70
calcium antagonists 41
calcium supplements 64, 67
capsulitis of shoulder 44, 83
captopril (Capoten) 41, 60
carbachol 101-2
carbamazepine (Tegretol) 111
   + amitryptiline (Tryptizol) 112

146

carcinoma of lung, hypertrophic osteoarthropathy due to 83
cardiac dysrhythmia 48–55
  aetiology 48–9
  classification 49
  investigation 50–2
  management 46, 52–5
cardiac failure 38
cardiogenic shock (circulatory collapse) 56
cardiovascular disease 3–4, 36
carotid endarterectomy 89
carpal tunnel syndrome 27, 110, 124
cataract 25
causes of disability/disease 7–8
cerebellar lesion 30
cerebrovascular accident 30
cerebrovascular insufficiency 27
chiropody 108
chlorambucil (Leukeran) 123
chlormethiazole (Heminevrin) 140, 142
chlorpromazine (Largactil) 21, 140
chlorpropamide (Diabenese) 133
chondrocalcinosis 82
chondrosarcoma 71
circulatory collapse (cardiogenic shock) 56
clomipramine (Anafranil) 142
cocaine 113
collapse 29–31
coma, drug-induced 30
community services 108–9
confusion 26–8
confusional state 27
Conn's syndrome 34
constipation 23–4
costochondritis (Teitz's syndrome) 45
cough 18–19
cough syncope 22
Coxsackie B myalgia (Bornholm disease) 45
cranial arteritis 89, 90
crystal synovitis 82–3

day hospital 109–10
decarboxylase inhibitor 94
dementia 28, 136–41
  epidemiology 4–5
  management 139
  multi-infarct (arteriosclerotic) 137
  presenile 28, 137
  RCP test (Hodkinson's modification) 139
  secondary 137
  senile 137
depression 5, 27, 28, 139, 141–2
diabetes mellitus 127–36
  aetiology 128

complications 129–31, 135
  management 131–6
diamorphine 58
diarrhoea 23–4
diazepam 140, 144
dichloralphenazone (Welldorm) 144
diclofenac (Voltarol) 77
digoxin 9, 46, 53, 58, 60, 126
  heart block due to 49
  intravenous 58
dihydroergot alkaloids 140
Diogenes syndrome 29, 119, 142–3
disodium etridonate (EHDP) 70
disopyramide (Norpace; Rythmodan) 46,
  54
district nursing service 104–5
diuretics 40
diverticulosis 24
drug compliance 9
drug interactions/unwanted effects 10
dyspnoea 16–18

elderly disabled 103–10
  aids for living/mobility 107
emepronium bromide (Cetiprin) 101
enalapril (Innovace) 41, 60
endocarditis, subacute bacterial 58
ephedrine 101
epidemiology 3–5
epilepsy 21, 30
essential thrombocythaemia 121–2
ethinyl oestradiol 65
exercise testing 45
extracranial-intracranial anastomosis 89
eyesight, failing 24–5

facet joint syndrome 113
faecal impaction 24, 26, 98, 99
faints, fits and falls 21–2
fibrositis (myofascial syndrome) 113
flavoxate (Urispas) 101
flecainide (Tambocor) 53, 54
folic acid deficiency 28, 118–19
frusemide (Lasix) 40, 46, 58, 59, 60

glaucoma 25
glibenclamide (Daonil) 133
glibornuride 133
glipizide 133
gliquidone 133
glyceryl trinitrate 58, 60
glymidine 133
'going off his feet' syndrome 20–1
goitre, non-toxic 127

gold therapy 77
golfer's elbow (medial epicondylitis) 83
gout 82-3
Graves' disease 28, 125

haloperidol (Serenace) 140
hearing loss 24, 25
heart block 49, 54
heart failure 55-60
    causes 56
    diagnosis 56-8
    investigation 56-8
    management 46, 58-60
Huntington's chorea 28, 137
hydralazine (Apresoline) 41, 60
hydrocephalus, normal pressure 94
hydrochlorothiazide (HydroSaluric) 40
    + amiloride (Moduretic) 59
hydroxycobalamin (Neo-Cytamen) 118
hyperglycaemia 29-30
hypertension 33-43
    aetiology 34
    assessment 38-9
    complications 35-8
    drug treatment 40-2
    investigation 39
    management 39-40
    planned care 42
    systolic 34
hyperthyroidism 28, 125-7
hypoglycaemia 29
hypoglycaemic agents 133
hypoproteinaemia 19-20
hypotensive states 22
hypothermia 27, 31
hypothyroidism (myxoedema) 27, 124-5

ibuprofen 70
imipramine (Tofranil) 101, 142
incontinence 25-6, 97-103
    aetiology 97-8
    appliances/catheters 102
    faecal 97, 102-3
    management 98-100, 102-3
    neurogenic 98, 100-2
    urinary 97
indomethacin (Indocid) 70, 77, 82
insulin 134
iodine, radioactive 126
iron sorbitol citrate (Jectofer) 117
ischaemic heart disease 43-8
    aetiology 43-4
    assessment 44-5
    complications 44

counselling 46-7
    investigation 44-5
    management 46
isosorbide dinitrate (Isordil) 47-8, 60
isoxsuprine (Duvadilan) 140
ispaghula (Fybogel; Metamucil) 98

joint replacement, rheumatoid arthritis 60

lactulose (Duphalac) 98
laevodopa 94-5
    + benserazide (Madopax) 94, 95
    + carbidopa (Sinemet) 94, 95
large bowel cancer 24
leucopaenia 123
leukaemia 122-3
local anaesthetic nerve block 112

management attitudes 8-9
Ménière's syndrome 25
mesothelioma of pleura 83
metabolic disease, epidemiology of 4
metformin (Glucophage) 133
methyl cellulose (Cologel; Celevac) 98
methyldopa 21
metoclopamide (Maxolon) 70
micturition syncope 22
misery 28-9
mithramycin (Mithracin) 70-1
morphine 58
mortality, observed/expected, at various ages
    38
multiple myeloma 72, 83
musculo-skeletal disease, epidemiology 4
myelofibrosis (myelosclerosis) 121
myeloproliferative syndrome 120-2
myocardial infarction 45
    cardiac arhythmias after 30
    management 46
    prevention of re-infarction 47
myofascial syndrome (fibrositis) 113
myxoedema (hypothyroidism) 27, 124-5

naftidrofuryl (Praxilene) 140
neuropathic arthropathy 83
neuropathy
    alcoholic 111
    autonomic 135
    diabetic 111, 130-1, 135
nifedipine (Adalat) 41, 48
nitrates 47-8, 58, 60
nitrazepam 144
non-steroidal anti-inflammatory drugs 70,
    74

organization of care 11–13
orphenadine (Disipal) 95, 140
osteitis deformans *see* Paget's disease
osteoarthritis 80–2
osteomalacia 23, 65–8, 112
osteoporosis 61–5
  aetiology 61–3
  differential diagnosis 63–4
  investigation 63–4
  management 64–5
  spinal vertebrae 112
osteosarcoma 71
oxprenolol 47

pacemakers 54–5
Paget's disease (osteitis deformans) 68–71
  aetiology 68
  differential diagnosis 69–70
  investigations 69–70
  management 70–1
pain 110–14
  malignant disease 113–14
  peripheral nerve injury, management 111–12
palpations 15–16
papillary muscle dysfunction 44
paraphrenia 27, 139
parkinsonism 91–7
  aetiology 92
  complications 93
  differential diagnosis 93–4
  drug-induced 92
  management 94–6
penicillamine 77
pericarditis 45
pethidine 113
phaeochromocytoma 34
phantom limb 111
phenformin 133
phenoxybenzamine (Dibenyline) 102
phenytoin (Epanutin) 111
physiotherapy 105–6
Pick's disease 28, 137
pindolol (Visken) 53
plantar fasciitis 83
poisoning 30–1
polycythaemia 120–1
polymyalgia rheumatica 23
population patterns 1–2
postherpetic neuralgia 110
posture, correct 105
prazosin (Hypovase) 21, 41
prednisolone 123
presbyacusis 25

prescribing principles 9–10
prevention of disability/disease 7–8
progressive supranuclear palsy (Steele-Richardson syndrome) 22, 93–4
promazine (Sparine) 140, 144
propranolol (Inderal) 40, 47, 48, 126
prostatic cancer 99–100, 113
prostatic hypertrophy 99
prostaglandin inhibitors 74
protryptilene (Concordin) 142
pseudogout 82
psychiatric disorders 136–42
pulmonary embolism 45

quinidine 53

reflux oesophagitis 45
reserpine 41
reticulum cell sarcoma 71
retinopathy, diabetic 129, 130
rheumatoid arthritis 74–80
  differential diagnosis 77
  investigation 76
  management 77–80

scurvy 119
selegiline hydrochloride (Eldepryl) 96
Shy-Drager syndrome 94
sick sinus syndrome 49, 54
sinus bradycardia 54
sleep problems 28–9, 143–4
social deprivation 28–9
social worker 108–9
sodium fluoride 112
speech therapy 108
spine, secondary deposits 23
spironolactone (Aldactone) 59–60
steal syndromes 69, 89
Steele-Richardson syndrome (progressive supranuclear palsy) 22, 93–4
steroids 77
  aplastic anaemia 123
  joint infection 79
  prostatic carcinoma 113
stilboestrol 73
strokes 84–91
  aetiology 84–5
  clinical features 85–6
  complications, early 87–8
  localization 86–7
  management 87–91
  prevention 89–90
suicide 31
subarachnoid haemorrhage 86

subclavian steal syndrome   89
sulphinpyrazone (Anturan)   47
supraspinatus tendinitis   83
swollen legs   19–20

tamoxifen   73
Teitz's syndrome (costochondritis)   45
temazepam (Euhypnos; Normison)   140, 144
temporal arteritis   25
tennis elbow (lateral epicondylitis)   83
thalamic pain   112
thioridazine (Melleril)   140
thyroid gland
  carcinoma   127
  disorders   124–7
thyroxine   125
timolol (Blocadren)   40, 47, 48
tocainide (Tonocard)   53
tolbutamide (Rastinon)   133
toxic confusional states   139
transcutaneous nerve stimulation (TENS)
    111, 112
transient ischaemic attacks   88–9
tremor
  benign essential   95

parkinsonian   92
  postural   96
triamterene (Dytac)   40, 59
trigeminal neuralgia   111
trinitrin   48

ulnar nerve compression   110

valvular rupture   58
vasodilators   41
vaso-vagal attacks   22
ventricular fibrillation   53
ventricular flutter   53
ventricular premature complexes   53
ventricular tachycardia   53
verapamil   53
vertebro-basilar ischaemia (insufficiency)
    89, 89–90
vitamin B_{12} deficiency   28
vitamin D   65, 65–6
vitamin D2   65
vitamin D3   65

Wolff–Parkinson–White syndrome   53